A
Woman's
Guide
to
Therapy

SUSAN STANFORD FRIEDMAN teaches English literature and women's studies at the University of Wisconsin-Madison.

LINDA GAMS teaches emotionally disturbed children.

NANCY GOTTLIEB is a writer and educator on health-care issues.

CINDY NESSELSON does vocational rehabilitation with mentally retarded and emotionally disturbed adults.

A Woman's Guide to Therapy

Susan Stanford Friedman

with coauthors
Linda Gams
Nancy Gottlieb
Cindy Nesselson

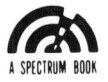

A SPECTRUM BOOK

Prentice-Hall, Inc., Englewood Cliffs, N.J. 07632

Library of Congress Cataloging in Publication Data

Friedman, Susan Stanford.
  A woman's guide to therapy.

  (A Spectrum Book)
  Bibliography: p.
  Includes index.
  1. Women—Mental health services.   2. Psychotherapy.
I. Title.
RC451.4.W6F75   362.2   78-32040
ISBN 0-13-961672-1
ISBN 0-13-961664-0 pbk.

RC
451.4
W6
F75

Editorial/production supervision
by Norma Miller Karlin
Interior design by Fred Dahl
and Norma Miller Karlin
Cover design by Muriel Nasser
Manufacturing buyer: Cathie Lenard

10 9 8 7 6 5 4 3 2 1

PRENTICE-HALL INTERNATIONAL, INC., *London*
PRENTICE-HALL OF CANADA, LTD., *Toronto*
PRENTICE-HALL OF INDIA PRIVATE LIMITED, *New Delhi*
PRENTICE-HALL OF JAPAN, INC., *Tokyo*
PRENTICE-HALL OF SOUTHEAST ASIA PTE. LTD., *Singapore*
WHITEHALL BOOKS LIMITED, *Wellington, New Zealand*

Contents

47265

Preface

WHAT WE DID; WHO WE ARE

This book may be of general interest to everybody, but it is particularly directed toward women who have been in therapy, women who are seeing a therapist now, or women who might turn to therapy for help at some time in the future. Our purpose is to give you some guidelines concerning what you can expect from most therapy, what you should look for in a therapist, and what kind of therapy you should avoid. Therapists are people too—the products of the same socializing processes that we experience and reflecting to varying degrees the values of the society at large. But when you're feeling worthless, inadequate, lonely, or helpless, it's hard to see beyond the immediate need to talk to someone who might help solve your problems. We have tried to imagine what you would face in deciding whether or not a therapist could help you. We have tried to suggest the questions you should ask, the kinds of attitudes you should watch out for, and the subtle assumptions the therapist might have about you as a woman—assumptions you might not be aware of because you're really upset. In short, what we're hoping is that we will give you a broader perspective from which you can evaluate your own therapist.

What this book has become after years of hard work, elation, discouragement, uncertainty, and a final pulling together is not exactly what we had in mind when we started. Perhaps you can evaluate the book better if you know something about us and all the various stages we went through in coming to this final point.

We were originally a group of six women who came together in 1971 during a women's studies course called "Alice in Academe" at the University of Wisconsin. At that time, we were between the ages of 19 and 28, from white, middle-class backgrounds. We were all heterosexual, and one was married with a young daughter. Three of us had had experience in therapy. None of us was a professional therapist or an "expert" in the field of psychology, although several of us had majored in psychology, one had worked as a summer intern at a mental hospital, and one had written a dissertation that dealt with Freud and Jung. After the first draft of this book was finished, three of us were involved in lay counseling for women and one was finishing an intern program for therapists.

We originally decided to evaluate psychological services in Madison because we had talked to women there who felt bitter and confused about their experiences with therapy. At first we thought that what would be most helpful to women thinking about therapy would be a list of local therapists whom we knew would not simply adjust a woman to an unjust society. But we couldn't make a list. First of all, the more we talked among ourselves about what makes a good therapist, the more we discovered that there was no single answer. No one set of criteria seemed to apply to everybody at all times and in all places. Second, even if we could have decided on criteria, we had no reliable way of rating therapists. We couldn't interview every therapist in town, and every questionnaire we tried to write seemed to make it too easy for the therapist to give the "right-sounding" answers.* So we decided to start by getting information we could be sure was accurate—concerning such things as cost, type of therapy, what happens at the first appointment, training of therapists in Madison. Then we would probe more indirect policies and problems. But this wasn't enough. Our concrete information would help a woman find a therapist and be confident that she knew what to expect, but it wouldn't help her avoid a destructive therapist.

In the process of designing a questionnaire and talking to therapists and to one another, we began to understand more clearly the general issues regarding women and therapy that our directory couldn't deal with. We felt something else was needed—not just another analysis or study of what therapists are like, but a guide written for women who actually have to face therapy for their own survival. The various chapters of the original tiny pamphlet grew bit by bit as we came to understand more and hear more from women willing to discuss their experiences.

The writing itself was also something of an experiment. Almost everything in the first draft was written jointly. The six of us would first discuss a subject together. Then two or three would be assigned that section. They would often talk out what needed to be said for hours before any writing started. Then one person wrote while the other(s) composed out loud. We didn't start out with this as a carefully plotted method. It just happened that way, until by the end it had become a really efficient and exciting way to work, to teach each other, and to share responsibility. Writing this way was

*Since we began meeting in 1971, information on specific therapists has been collected in Madison. We know that lists of both destructive and helpful therapists are being made all over the country now. If you want a specific referral, try calling a local Women's Center or a local chapter of the National Organization of Women.

something completely new for all of us. We felt liberated from the procrastinating problems of trying to write alone. The experience of talking and producing together changed us all.

This collective stage of work was interrupted in 1973, just after we completed our first draft, because people graduated and moved to other parts of the country. The physical separation and the differing requirements of our work lives succeeded in ending our original group effort. Since then, the book has gone through several more stages. Two women eventually dis-associated themselves from the effort because they felt it didn't go deeply enough into the *economic* causes of women's unhappiness. One of us went over the first draft to rewrite, unify, and synthesize the various parts. New sections were added where gaps in subject matter seemed to be serious flaws. Interviews with ex–mental patients made possible a greatly expanded section on mental institutions. Then one of us took all the interview material from Madison psychiatric services to shape voluminous data into a coherent case study of different types of institutions. And another did a final stylistic editing job on the second draft. All of this work was done individually, the original collective style of writing having been abandoned out of necessity.

Four of us returned to work together to complete yet another stage of revision needed to submit the manuscript for publication. And finally one of us took on the responsibility of final rewriting. The book therefore has resulted from a combination of work done jointly and separately. Yet, however important the individual efforts were, it was clear to everyone that the energy and framework of ideas and questions had come from the collective phase of the work.

Many people have helped our project by reading, criticizing, and showing enthusiasm for what we wrote and by sharing their own experience with us. We would particularly like to thank Nancy Henley, whose thoughtful comments gave us the incentive to revise and prepare the manuscript for publication. We are grateful to the people of the New

England Free Press, who gave us a very fine critical reading and encouraged us to continue our efforts. The writers who have published in the *Radical Therapist* (later *Rough Times,* and currently *State and Mind*) were a great source of information and inspiration. We also appreciate the help of Nicole Anthony, Robert Badesch, Margery Barnet, Evelyn T. Beck, Barbara Bitters, Ruth Bjork, Ellie Budow, Neal Cariello, Victoria Cazel, Bonnie Freeman, Mary Frey, Edward Friedman, Jane Friedman, Diane Gottlieb, Maureen Green, Cathy Greenspan, Lisa Hunter, Ruth Ice, Carol Jackson, Irene Javors, Diane Kravetz, Evelyn Machtinger, Betty Maher, Roy Okada, Sandra O'Leary, Elaine Reuben, Sonia Rogers, Barbara Rothberg, Judy Sanders, Lee Scheingold, Louise Scott, Julia Sherman, Mary Waters, and Karen Wick.

A
Woman's
Guide
to
Therapy

Women and Therapy: The Problems, Realities, and Potentials

For what reasons do women seek therapy? Can therapy help women who feel they cannot handle their problems alone? What are some of the unique problems women are likely to encounter in therapy? There are many factors that influence the way therapists (men *and* women) view and treat women— not the least of which is the way women have been socialized to see *themselves*. The reality is that today therapy is not necessarily a helpful, constructive process for women in emotional pain. Why is this? And what must occur in the practice of therapy as well as in people's ways of thinking to make therapy a viable aid to women who need help? These are some of the questions and issues we will address in this chapter.

THE WOMAN WHO SEEKS THERAPY

When a lover leaves, or when a marriage fails, or when children leave home, a woman's loneliness may become unbearable. When she feels ugly, or isn't having orgasms, or faces menopause or hysterectomy, a woman may begin to doubt that she's a "real woman." When she feels inferior to everyone else, or when boredom and restlessness reach a peak, or when there is a feeling that her life may have been worthless, a woman may become trapped in self-hatred, fearing the emptiness of the future. When she feels guilty about her sexuality, or fears success, or believes she is too "aggressive," a woman may find herself torn between what she really is and what she thinks she "should" be.

It's at times like these that many women turn to therapy. In this country, therapy has become a massive socially sanctioned institution that exists for the purpose of "curing" unhappiness, anxiety, or depression. And women are seeking help from this growing institution in great numbers. In fact, women outnumber men in out-patient therapy, including both clinic and private settings. One authority asserts that anywhere between 60 percent to 75 percent of all people in therapy are women; and the number of women turning to therapy is increasing at a higher rate than the number of men.[1]

Women generally enter therapy with tremendous feelings of inadequacy and self-hatred, with self-destructive thoughts and sometimes actions. (The number of suicide attempts is much higher among women than men; men more often turn their anger toward others.[2]) Women are guilt-ridden and blame themselves for their unhappiness; thus they often turn their resentment against themselves. People around them tend to see them as failures. They see themselves as failures. And the result is depression, anxiety, and self-loathing. Pauline Bart's interviews with middle-aged women hospitalized for depression illustrate vividly the sense of inadequacy and emptiness that affects many women, particularly those whose role as mother and wife has decreased in value as youth vanishes and children leave home. One woman told Bart:

> I don't—I don't—I don't feel like[d].—I don't feel that I'm wanted. I don't feel at all that I'm wanted. I just feel like nothing. I don't feel

anybody cares, and nobody's interested, and they don't care whether I do feel good or I don't feel good. I'm pretty useless . . . I feel like I want somebody to feel for me, but nobody does.[3]

Another woman told Bart how the needs of her daughter kept her functioning; when her children were gone, however, her feelings of identity and self-worth collapsed:

But in the morning I would get up, and I knew that there was so much dependent on me, and I didn't want my daughter to become depressed about it or neurotic in any way, which could have easily happened because I had been that way. So I'm strong-minded and strong-willed, so I would pull myself out of it. It's just recently that I couldn't pull myself out of it. I think that if there was—if I was needed maybe I would have, but I feel that there's really no one that needs me now.[4]

This kind of negative identity parallels the self-hate evident in minority people who have internalized the barrage of stereotypes from the dominant culture. Minority sub-cultures—Black, Puerto Rican, Chicano, Asian-American, Native American, Jewish, etc.—have countered this stereotyping by creating positive images and identities based on racial and cultural pride. While the women's movement has had some effect in its attack on traditional norms for femininity and the devaluation of women, many troubled women today continue to see their problems as unique, as *personal* inadequacies. Because women are often isolated from the suffering of other women (women seldom reveal the full extent of their "failures" to other women), many do not understand that their problems are shared by other women. Unaware of the comprehensive social problems underlying their individual sense of failure, women often do not see the origin of their problems in the societal norms and institutions that greatly restrict acceptable behavior for women.

Many women share common difficulties—but each one has her own way of dealing or not dealing with the restrictions of her environment. But a woman isn't likely to be helped if she and her therapist do not understand that the ultimate source of many problems is not an idiosyncratic childhood or character. The origin is *first* in the culture itself—that culture which so narrowly defines the primary role for a woman as loving wife and mother—and *second* in the social and economic institutions that block or make difficult any woman's attempt to break out of the traditional mold. According to the norms of society, learned by each young girl from the media, books, toys, her environment in general and sometimes her parents in particular, a woman's worth and identity is ultimately defined by the man she is with, by the children she produces, by the image she projects, by the ingenuity of her home-making, and by the uncomplaining grace with which she fulfills the expectations attached to these roles.

Here's a telling Jewish folktale, quoted by Bart:

> A young man begs his mother for her heart, which a betrothed of his has demanded as a gift; having torn it out of his mother's proffered breast, he races away with it; and as he stumbles, the heart falls to the ground, and he hears it question protectively, "Did you hurt yourself, my son?"[5]

Although many women, as well as men, have internalized these norms, few women can adjust to them with any real success. Many women who have accepted marriage and children as their most important goal are still finding their lives to be desperately unhappy. Women who have been able to reject this limited role in part are nonetheless confronted with a society that considers them "misfits" or "maladjusted." Many either suffer greatly from the pressures of being different or develop guilt feelings about their reluctance or inability to be satisfied with living only through others. Most women accept the socially imposed view that it is up to *them* to change if things are going wrong.

A woman married to a physician wrote a letter to a medical journal that succinctly expresses this common cultural belief that the wife's *responsibility* in marriage is to keep the marriage going while the husband's duty is to provide the money and social prestige. The journal, *Medical Economics*, had run a column by a psychiatrist, Dr. Thomas P. Hackett, called "Can You Handle the Medical Man's Menopause?" He was answering the troubled letter from a woman whose middle-aged physician husband had lost all interest in his work and marriage. Hackett's article described the symptoms of male menopause and suggested some possible remedies, including therapy for the physician. His article touched off a flood of mail from male doctors and medical wives, all blaming the troubled wife for the "medical man's menopause." One woman wrote:

> Let me tell you wives . . . that your influence in marriage is unlimited. Men do not like to change the status quo unless it becomes absolutely untenable. Your life together can be exciting and rewarding right up to the very last years. But the one who makes it that way must be *you*. And you don't just let it happen—it takes a lot of work. If you are running into any trouble in your marriage, or you see signs that the male bird in your nest is getting restless or depressed or unhappy in any way, don't try to influence him to see a psychiatrist: Go yourself![6]

Many women do indeed enter therapy because their husband's problems have been a predominant factor in the disintegration of a marriage. Many other women guiltily internalize their husband's and children's failures as their own and become deeply depressed or self-deprecating. This blame that Kay Wright so cheerfully consigns to wives is destructive. The real "culprit," we believe, is *not* the woman, but her situation. The more a woman has internalized the dominant cultural norms, the more she will blame herself for her problems and misunderstand the role of her situation in establishing severe psychological strain.

It is the isolation of being trapped in a home with no car and only toddlers to talk to that drives many young women to depression and paralysis—*not* their failure to be loving mothers. And it *is* the culture's disapproval of independent women that stands behind many working women's anxiety about success in traditionally defined "masculine" roles—*not* their failure to be "real women." It *is* the widespread fear of homosexuality (homophobia) that causes many lesbian women to distrust their own sexual orientation—*not* "mental illness" produced by family relationships in early childhood. It *is* a genuine role loss and the destructive youth-orientation of American culture that leads some middle-aged homemakers to a lonely alcoholism after their children leave home—*not* "neurotic" tendencies in their psychological makeup.

Response to society's sometimes velvet (and sometimes not-so-velvet) cage varies greatly—all the way from mild depression to suicide. Each woman copes with the pressures of her own and others' expectations in her own way. But unless it is understood what role those expectations play in the creation and intensification of her problems, that lonely, anxious, self-deprecating woman is not likely to change her unhappiness.

THE THERAPIST

We've looked at some of the reasons why women seek therapy; now let's look at the therapists themselves. An overwhelming majority of therapists are male and white—90 percent of practicing psychiatrists and 67 percent of clinical psychologists, according to some statistics.[7] In recent years, more women have asked for women therapists, but anyone who has specifically requested a woman therapist knows how difficult it is to find one with free time. But whether the therapist is male or female, he or she shares a common psychological training and personal upbringing in a world that rigidly divides the sexes.

The Influence of Stereotypes

Emerging almost inevitably from the therapist's professional and individual background are certain stereotypes about women that are bound to enter directly or subliminally into therapy sessions.

Sometimes these stereotypes affect therapy in a very overt way. For example, one professional woman recalled her experience with a Jungian therapist when she was at an important crossroads of her life. She was an aspiring poet with a great urge to create. Her therapist told her straightforwardly that women can experience the exhilaration of creation by having babies. She should have a child, he advised, and her desire to create would be fulfilled. Such value-laden recommendations in therapy are often easy to spot simply because they are so very blatant.

However, sometimes a therapist's assumptions about appropriate identities and roles for women are very subtle and even subconscious. The power of such assumptions to color and direct the perceptions of even the best-intentioned therapists is enormous. To illustrate how difficult it is for a woman in therapy to identify these hidden norms and how potentially harmful they can be, we present, with the author's permission, a condensed account of Claire Pomeroy's experience, recorded in her published diary of her therapy, *Fight It Out, Work It Out, Love It Out, The Story of a Family in Therapy*[8]:

Claire and Adam had been going to a fine therapist for many weeks; they trusted him, liked him, and felt at home with his values. He was well known in the area as a nontraditional therapist; he even had a poster on his wall from a group of therapists who were challenging the mainstream ideas of their profession. Consequently, he was deeply aware of how socialization could enter into people's problems. But one day he told the couple that he wanted to be honest with them; he wanted to tell them what he had been thinking about them (he didn't pretend to be objective or noninvolved). To Adam he said, "I like you very much. I feel very comfortable with you, as if we had been special friends for years. The main reason for my good feeling is that we have shared an intellectual thing together; I really feel close to you because of all the ideas we have discussed and the importance our work has for each of us." To Claire he said, "You are a warm, beautiful, loving person, but I don't feel really comfortable with you. I feel we don't really connect—there is a barrier between us. It comes from the fact that you are keeping a diary of these sessions, that there is this intellectual part of you, separate from the rest, that is reflecting on everything and writing it down. I like Claire the Woman, but I am uncomfortable with Claire the Writer. The Writer part of you is keeping me from having a warm relationship with you."

Adam agreed with the therapist. Suddenly, there were two men lined up against her, saying that her womanly potential was blocked by her mind. She was very upset, practically speechless, furious, but unable to defend herself for several weeks. Later she began insisting that the Writer and the Woman were the same person, that the therapist felt close to Adam because of their intellectual life and distant from her because of hers. Neither Adam nor the therapist would accept what she said—they kept insisting that she was two different people. She began working out her anger by writing up a description of the past few sessions; the profound sexism of the therapist became clearer to her and she withdrew from the therapy, showing him what she had written. He was angry at first, and very hurt, but he finally admitted to both Claire and Adam that he was chauvinist and sexist.

Like the rest of us, therapists are human beings who grew up in the world as it is; and like us, they have not escaped the influence of traditional views on what a woman should be.

Let's assume that your therapist is a man who has expected his wife to take over full responsibilities in their home. He provides for the family; she clothes, feeds, and nurtures the family while he (and perhaps she) resists any idea that she might leave the home to get a job. It would take a nearly hopeless, certainly conscious, effort for this man to prevent his personal expectations of women from playing some part in his expectations of you and his analysis of your problems.

Or suppose your therapist is a single woman who in her own life has had to be more committed, harder-working, and better qualified than male therapists to make it in her profession. Particularly if she grew up in the thirties or forties, she probably had to make a choice between career and family. This inhuman choice not imposed on men was frequently assumed for women at a time when combining a job and family was even less acceptable for middle-class women than it is today. Her feelings about that choice and the pressures on her to be a superprofessional are bound to affect your therapy—especially if you are struggling to have both a family and a job, or if you are fighting weakness, passivity, and lack of self-confidence in your work. Her own prejudices can be as harmful to you as those of a male therapist.

One young woman told us:

> *I went to see a woman therapist because I was 30 pounds overweight and I felt I had no friends. My therapist was a woman, and she was very domineering, always telling me what I should do, never really listening to me. One day, I told her she was acting just like my mother, and that my mother bossing me around might have had something to do with why I am so fat. She said, "I knew it all along. I was just waiting for you to blame it all on your mother." She told me she had called up my mother without my knowing it and had talked to her about my problems. She said, "I want you to go home and work things out with your mother. Nobody can help you with your problems until you do. If you don't settle things with her, you'll probably be fat forever."*

The Influence of Psychological Theories

Intensifying whatever private notions the therapist has about what a woman should be are his or her *psychological theories* about what is healthy behavior for women. These theories have rarely questioned the traditional view that men and women are inherently different or that the division of labor reflected in acceptable male and female roles is justifiable or inevitable. And *most psychological schools see people's problems emerging from individual hang-ups rather than from basic injustices in the society as a whole.* Professional training often just reinforces the influence of the personal background of therapists, adding the stamps of Authority, Science, and Truth to private opinion and general custom. Your therapist will most likely deny being a proponent of any particular school (therapists we interviewed always told us they were "eclectic") but the reading on women they did while in training is bound to have had some influence.

Some of the important theorists of twentieth-century psychology are likely to have had a significant influence on any therapist's education. Many of these writers have very explicit theories on the psychology of women that can potentially reinforce your therapist's personal beliefs. For example, Hélèn Deutsch, a disciple of Freud, wrote:

> The essentially sound activity and the social and intellectual energy developed by the young girl who renounces her fantasies often blights her emotional life and prevents her from achieving complete femininity and later motherhood.[9]

And Erik Erikson wrote:

> Young women often ask whether they can "have an identity" before they know whom they will marry and for whom they will make a home. Granted that something in the young woman's identity must keep itself open for the peculiarities of the man to be joined and of the children to be brought up, I think that much of a young woman's identity is already defined in her kind of attractiveness and in the selectivity of her search for the man (or men) by whom she wishes to be sought.[10]

The Broverman study, done on therapists themselves, confirms our conviction that training and background have made therapists see normal behavior for women and men as fundamentally different. On the Broverman questionnaire, there was *no* difference in the way male and female therapists responded. For what they considered "healthy" qualities in men, most of them checked off "very aggressive," "very independent," "very dominant," "not at all emotional," "likes math and science," "very competitive," "very logical," "almost always acts as a leader," "never conceited about appearance," "very ambitious," "never cries," and so forth. For what they considered "healthy" qualities in women, most of them marked "very tactful," "very neat," "very gentle," "very quiet," "very strong need for security," "very interested in own appearance," "easily expresses tender feelings," and so forth. When sex was not designated, they equated "healthy" behavior with all the qualities they had previously assigned *to men.* In other words, behavior considered "healthy" for a woman appears to be considered neurotic or unhealthy for a human being. So a large majority of therapists today has different standards of mental health for women than for men—standards that they still see as negative for human beings.[11]

The Influence of the Environment

Because so many therapists have not questioned the influence of stereotypes and psychological theories on therapy for women, they often do not understand fully what role a woman's environment plays in creating or intensifying problems. Like women themselves, therapists tend to see problems as unique, as arising out of personal failures to cope with the world. They are likely to try to help women *adjust* to this environment rather than helping them *change* their situations. In seeking to free women from their problems and push them in the direction of individual fulfillment, therapists are all too likely to urge a discretion consistent with their own notion of what fulfillment means for a woman.

An examination of Freud's description of his work with a young paralyzed girl illustrates the typical therapist's attempts to adjust women to traditional roles, sometimes with disastrous consequences. In his essay "Analysis Terminable and Interminable," Freud was exploring the question of how long analysis must last to be effective. He told the story of a young girl who came to him for help concerning sudden paralysis of her legs. After analysis, she walked again, and in the face of terrible family fortunes she proved to be the rock of stability for her disheartened parents. But when she was 25, facing a hysterectomy and the prospect of bearing no children, she had another breakdown from which she never recovered. Freud concluded that her initial analysis hadn't been long enough.[12] But might there not be another explanation? Perhaps Freud, acting on his own and his culture's definition of what a woman should be, constructed an identity for the girl that made motherhood necessary. Perhaps without children, the girl felt worthless—all her sense of self collapsed, and her breakdown became complete.

This kind of therapy does not bring about permanent solutions to women's depressions, anxieties, or suicide attempts; instead, it effects a temporary adjustment to the limited expectations and possibilities for women. On the whole, therapy has become an institution which—whatever its stated goals, whatever the good intentions of its therapists—*helps keep women in their place.*

THE POTENTIAL FOR THERAPY

Given this overall impact of therapy on most women, is there any positive potential for therapy? It is our belief that the problems women face because of sexism will not disappear until restrictive societal norms affecting women are changed. Traditional therapy, which tends to reinforce those norms of the status quo, can provide no real solution. In order for women to change and grow in therapy, therapists themselves must also undergo some changes. They need to re-evaluate the sex-role biases of their professional training and to recognize what assumptions they have unconsciously been making about the psychology of women. Only in this way can a therapist begin to deal with women rather than roles, with human beings rather than images. Only in this way can an atmosphere be created in therapy which can help a woman expand her self-image and gain the strength to confront the constrictive expectations and institutions that surround her.

But this change on the part of therapists and women is only a beginning. Therapy has developed as an institution that deals with the feelings of inadequacy that the culture has ingrained in women. At its best, therapy can help women realize that their problems are not inevitably the result of individual failure, but more likely the result of how an oppressive society has "failed" them as women. Therapy does have the potential of liberating women from paralyzing guilt and self-hatred. It can help women to understand the destructive effects of the system on their lives, to explore new identities, and to develop the confidence to challenge that system in both their private and public worlds.

Individual change, however, is not the equivalent of wide-scale systemic change. The woman who has forged a new, stronger identity through therapy must still confront institutional discrimination and limiting cultural norms. By itself, even nontraditional therapy cannot change laws, economic systems, or political structures. It is important to understand that unless the institutions that restrict women change, therapy can be at best only a patchwork job. It is even more important to realize that many women in the United States (as well as in the rest of the world) do not have access to *any* therapy at all. For poor women struggling to maintain basic survival, fulfillment is a luxury and therapy an impossibility.

We believe, therefore, that therapy does have the potential to help some women, but that it can never be a cure-all for the psychological and institutional problems women face. It cannot take the place of political action against the conditions that shape women's lives. It can contribute to, but not substitute for women coming together in a wide variety of ways to share their newly discovered anger, strength, and creative energy. And side by side with other organizations dedicated to social change, therapy can potentially play a significant role in helping that change come about.

Will therapy always be necessary? Perhaps if society can ever rid itself of discriminatory practices against *all* women, generalized feelings of inadequacy will not be common to most women. The need for many women to seek therapy might then be greatly diminished. Yes, individual differences would still exist; problems would still exist. But the intensity of these problems would lessen if women were able to function within a supportive living situation. For many, the *one* and *only* therapist would no longer be needed—PEOPLE WOULD HAVE EACH OTHER.

FOOTNOTES

[1]See Saul V. Levine, Louisa E. Kamin, Eleanor Lee Levine, "Sexism and Psychiatry," *American Journal of Orthopsychiatry*, 44, no. 3 (April 1974), 329–30. See also Phyllis Chesler's statistics in "Patient and Patriarch: Women in the Psychotherapeutic Relationship" in *Woman in Sexist Society*, Vivian Gornick and Barbara K. Moran, eds. (New York: Basic Books, 1971), pp. 364–70.

[2]Ibid., p. 329

[3]Pauline Bart, "Mother Portnoy's Complaints," *Transaction*, Vol. 8, no. 1–2 (November–December, 1970), p. 71. Published by permission of Transaction, Inc., from *Transaction*, Vol. 8, #1–2, Copyright © 1970 by Transaction, Inc. Since its original publication as "Mother Portnoy's Complaints," Bart's article has been widely anthologized under the title "Depression in Middle-Aged Women." See Vivian Gornick and Barbara K. Moran, eds., *Woman in Sexist Society* (New York: Basic Books, 1971), pp. 163–86.

[4]Ibid., p. 70.

[5]Ibid., p. 69.

[6]Quoted in "Who's Usually to Blame for the Medical Man's Menopause? His Wife!" *Medical Economics*, 49, no. 2 (June 19, 1972), 80.

[7]Saul V. Levine, Louisa E. Kamin, Eleanor Lee Levine, "Sexism and Psychiatry," *American Journal of Orthopsychiatry*, 44, no. 3 (April 1974), 329.

[8]From *Fight It Out, Work It Out, Love It Out*, by Claire Pomeroy. Copyright © 1977 by Doubleday & Company, Inc. Reprinted by permission of the publisher. The entire account, including the conversation in quotes, is paraphrased from the book with permission of the author and publisher.

[9]Hélène Deutsch, *The Psychology of Women*, Vol. I (New York: Grune & Stratton, 1944), pp. 127–28; see also Germaine Greer's discussion of Deutsch in *The Female Eunuch* (New York: Bantam Books, 1970), p. 95.

[10]Erik Erikson, "Inner and Outer Space: Reflections on Womanhood," *Daedalus*, 93 (1964), 582–606; see also Phyllis Chesler's comments on Erikson in "Patient and Patriarch: Women in the Therapeutic Relationship," in Gornick and Moran, *Woman in Sexist Society*, p. 378.

[11]Inge K. Broverman and Donald Broverman et al., "Sex-Role Stereotypes and Clinical Judgments of Mental Health," *Journal of Consulting and Clinical Psychology*," 34, no. 1 (1970), 1–7.

[12]Sigmund Freud, "Analysis Terminable and Interminable" (1937), trans. Joan Riviere, in *Therapy and Technique*, Philip Rieff, ed. (New York: Macmillan, 1963), p. 240.

The Decision to Seek Therapy

How do women make the decision to see a therapist? What kinds of attitudes do women have about therapy before they actually experience it? The answers cover an enormous range of expectations and states of mind.

Some women experiencing a tremendous crisis in their life seek therapy so they can get through the difficult period. Other recognize certain negative patterns in their behavior and see therapy as a means of self-exploration and possible change. Some make an appointment to see a therapist believing that just one session will help; others enter therapy certain that they will need long-term analysis.

Many women turn to a therapist when they are having marriage problems.* Other women are thrust into some type of therapy by the courts or some governmental agency. Some

---

*People are likely to assume that if a relationship is troubled, it is the *wife* who should go into therapy, since her major responsibility is considered to be the maintenance of smooth relationships in the home.

women already have a comprehensive intellectual under-standing of their problems, but seek therapy because their feelings and behavior are not in tune with what their intellect tells them. Many women hope that a therapist can help them decide "what to do" with the rest of their life. And for some women, therapy appears to be a safe arena in which confusions about sexuality, gender identity, and sex roles can be explored.

On the grimmer side, many women experience such severe depression, anxiety, and guilt that they are literally driven to seek therapy. They may be extremely lonely, physically or emotionally cut off from family or other supportive groups. This isolation can easily initiate a vicious circle that leaves therapy as the only recourse, because depression is so often accompanied by emotional withdrawal and dissociation from potential friends. Some of these women have spent hours obsessively considering suicide, and may seek therapy as a final avenue of help. Utter despair, uncontrolled or frightening behavior, and attempted suicide all bring women to therapy.

Women's attitudes toward therapy are often deeply influenced by the experiences and beliefs of friends and family. As common as therapy is today, many women are ashamed to go to a therapist—it seems to be an open admission of failure, or even worse, of "mental illness." Fear, distrust, and suspicion are also common attitudes, especially when a woman has known someone else who has had a bad experience in therapy. Some women are extremely guarded with a therapist for a long time; on the other hand, some are immediately trusting, certain that the therapist can provide all the necessary answers. Some decide easily to go into therapy, and others agonize for months over the decision.

Chances are that you may recognize yourself in one of these descriptions. In this chapter, we will examine some aspects of therapy that may affect your own decision and attitude about therapy. But first, for you who might be particularly anguished and desperate, we have a special comment to make.

A SPECIAL WORD TO WOMEN IN DESPAIR

Some of us who have worked on this book know from personal experience your despair, your sense that there is no place to turn, your feeling that nothing you do will lead to any resolution. You may feel that if you can't find help somewhere, you will "go crazy," or withdraw from life entirely; you may believe that things will never be different, or that you will have to go to a mental institution, or that eventually you might kill yourself. Therapy may seem to you to be your last chance—the only alternative, the only way you can possibly bring about a change. Although this book continually warns of the difficulties and dangers involved in therapy, this does not mean we are trying to take away your last straw of hope. Therapy can be one route to strength, dignity, and growth—particularly if you choose your therapist carefully. The most important advice we offer is that you *not* go to a therapist to lay your suffering, with unquestioning trust, at the feet of a miracle worker. Therapists are not gods and they are not always right. You need to go into therapy with critical intelligence and some willingness to trust the validity of your *own* feelings, no matter how much you hate yourself. Not all therapists will automatically be good for *you*. Take your time in choosing a therapist. Shop around, ask some questions, be critical. All our warnings are directed toward helping you become aware of possible dangers so you can select a therapist more wisely and evaluate what your therapist says to you about yourself.

Particularly if you are afraid you may try to kill yourself, this advice might seem somewhat general. More concretely, you could try any of the following:

1. Call a women's center or the local chapter of the National Organization for Women in your area and ask if it has a list of recommended therapists. Even if you have never gone to a women's center, the people there will be glad to refer you. If you live near a college or university with a women's studies program, those in charge may be able to give you some names.

2. Look in the Yellow Pages, or in the back of any feminist magazine, such as *Ms.*, to see if a feminist referral service exists near you. This service can provide names of therapists. Some of these referral collectives are listed in the back of this book.

3. Try to plan things so you won't be alone with nothing to do and no one to talk to for long stretches of time. Keep in touch with a friend or even an acquaintance who might be able to help you locate the kind of help you need.

4. Try to restrain yourself from latching on to the first therapist you can find. You will be much better off if you can look upon the first session or two as "interviews" in which you will decide whether or not the therapist is suitable for you.

5. Remember that there are many alternatives open to you—there are many possibilities that lie between the extremes of getting *no* help and of going into a mental hospital. Especially if you are at some crisis point in your life or you have just tried to commit suicide, a mental institution might be the worst place you could go for help. Many cities and counties have halfway houses or clinics where you can live for a short period of time. Even a short stay in a regular hospital is an option, a place where you can be "safe" with yourself. Find out what is available in your area.

THE PURPOSE OF THERAPY: ADJUSTMENT OR CHANGE?

If you are in therapy now or thinking about it, you are probably discontented with yourself and your life and hope a therapist can show you some way out of your maze of problems. But this raises several important questions about the kinds of solutions therapy may offer. Will the aim of your therapy be to ease your unhappiness by teaching you to adjust to the situation that made you unhappy in the first place —that is, will it teach you to accommodate yourself to the people around you and to their expectations of you? Or will therapy help you change your situation and create a new life for yourself—one that is not thwarted by the status quo? This issue of adjustment versus change is particularly crucial if your dissatisfactions relate in any way to the expectations society, family, and friends have for you *as a woman*. If therapy is primarily adjustment-oriented, it will teach you how to accept your role as woman, helpmate, and mother. If therapy encourages change, it may offer you a way to deal with the cultural and economic constrictions on you as a woman so that you can struggle toward an identity of your own choosing. By itself, therapy, because of its emphasis on individuals, can't liberate you from those constrictions, but at best it can give you some support in your efforts to break out of traditional molds.

Therapy as Adjuster

In actual practice, therapy has been used primarily as an adjuster. Women have often been encouraged to dissolve their anger, adapt to their situation as an unchangeable given, and redirect their dissatisfaction into "constructive" energy that can make them ever better mothers, wives, and lovers. This message from much therapy has been deeply reinforced by the general media image of women's dissatisfaction as selfish and their anger as ridiculous or hysterical. Persuasively suggesting that anger will be futile, the culture in many ways often subtly suggests that smiles and laughter will make women more acceptable. And many therapists reinforce this idea.

If you suspect your therapist of encouraging a "laughing slave" mentality, try the "turnaround test." Imagine you are a man—would your therapist give you the same advice or analysis of the situation? Or would he/she insist that you should not put up with your situation any longer?

Recommendations of adjustment are understandable, given some of the fundamental assumptions of psychology that have evolved since Freud. Psychology has been the study of *individual* behavior. And most psychologists have understood all human interaction by isolating the individual rather than by looking at the impact of societal divisions into groups (sex, class, race) on the development of the individual. Psychologists analyze the problems we face in terms of personal failure instead of in terms of society's inadequacies. The blame is placed squarely on our shoulders, and we are expected to cure our "deviances" by adjusting to a standard of normal behavior. "Sickness," "mental illness," "craziness" are seen as belonging to the individual and not to society. The whole concept of "mental illness" assumes that adjustment to the world as it is constitutes "mental health." Anyone dissatisfied with the status quo is by definition "maladjusted."

Susan Dworkin Levering summed up the prevailing definitions of insanity and sanity in her article that is critical of traditional therapy:

> *"Crazy"* is when a woman doesn't want to live with her husband any more. "Sane" is when she decides to wear a skirt and apply for a job at Bell Telephone.[1]

Freud's idea was that sickness or neurosis was personal, the inability of the individual to adapt to her (or his) environment, what he called the "real world." Anyone rebelling against the "real world" was operating on illusions or delusions—they were, in short, "crazy."

Psychology has in many ways repudiated many of Freud's theories, but his basic assumption—that what is "healthy," "normal," "sane," and "real" is what is accepted or approved of by society—still pervades much of modern clinical psychology. And what this means for women is that psychology tends to prescribe for its women "patients" the traditional woman's role.

Levering illustrates this in her description of two women in a state mental institution:

> Madeline is in her late thirties. The first time she was hospitalized her husband had her committed because she was neglecting her appearance and refused to have sexual relations with him. Of course she had been seriously depressed following the birth of her 3 children and didn't want to become pregnant again.
>
> Cathy is in her early twenties. Her parents had her committed when she wrote to them saying that she was going to find her own life with her own values. The admission records give as reasons for her hospitalization: hippie-type appearance, masculine attire (jeans and boots), sexual acting-out (sleeping with men she wasn't married to) and being unable to find her place in life despite finishing college.[2]

Since psychology seldom takes into consideration the limitations of cultural and social forces on women, it seldom understands the possibilities of their freedom. If we can begin to see some of our problems as relating to all women, we will stop blaming ourselves—stop hating ourselves—for what we used to see as personal failures. Once we begin to understand what social forces are creating problems for us, we can stop turning our energies against ourselves and start directing those energies toward the development of the strength and self-confidence necessary for pushing back against the forces of a difficult society. Real change, not just adjustment, becomes a possibility.

How do these assumptions of psychology relate to what happens between you and your therapist? If your therapist accepts the traditional conceptions of women—which all of us have grown up with in our culture and which greatly affect the training of therapists—then chances are that his/her desire to make you a fully functioning human being will translate into an attempt to make you a "warm, loving wife and mother"—and nothing more. Your therapist will try to get you to understand your unhappiness and discontent as your inability to totally fulfill yourself through your role. Even if he/she is aware you have other potential abilities as well, there may be an assumption that adjustment to the traditional role of women is easiest and will make you happiest. The women's movement has been quite successful in recent years in getting many people, including some therapists, to rethink their assumptions about sex roles. But profound social change comes slowly, with the consequence that many seeming changes cover up deep-seated traditional beliefs that go "underground" into subliminal layers of consciousness. Many therapists today would not define successful therapy for women and men in the categorically traditional terms that Freud and his colleague Ferenczi used:

> ... in every male patient the sign that his castration-anxiety has been mastered must be forthcoming, and this sign is a sense of equality of rights with the analyst; and every female patient, if her cure is to rank as complete and permanent, must have finally conquered her masculinity-complex and become able to submit without bitterness to thinking in terms of her feminine role.[3]

But similar assumptions of successful therapy as passive acceptance of a "feminine role" may subtly shape the perspectives of many a more "liberal" therapist.

If you have already questioned society's limited expectations of you as a woman (whether or not you are involved in the women's movement), you already know that this attitude that you must "submit" or adjust to the feminine role is destructive. If you have the self-confidence to speak out, your sessions with your therapist are likely to lead to open warfare. If you disagree on such fundamental issues, you will probably never be able to get anywhere with your therapist. If you don't have the confidence to openly question your therapist's assumptions about women, what confidence you do have may slowly be eaten away as you listen to your therapist's opinions and indirect suggestions without being able to respond. Eventually you may begin doubting the validity of your original dissatisfactions and end up feeling more worthless than when you started out.

If you don't think that your problems relate to your identity as a woman, or if you happily accept the cultural norms as your destiny, then the therapist can play a more subtly destructive role. You may be very willing to accommodate yourself to his/her idea of how a woman is fulfilled, and you and your therapist may consider the therapy successful. But if your problems relate to your being a woman, then that "adjustment" which you and your therapist have so carefully created may eventually fall to pieces. Because the therapist has neither eliminated any of the outside pressures on you nor given you the strength to fight them, old problems may return, perhaps in new forms.

One depressed middle-aged woman told Pauline Bart:

> I'm glad that God gave me . . . the privilege of being a mother . . . and I loved [my children]. In fact, I wrapped my love so much around them. . . . I'm grateful to my husband since if it wasn't for him, there wouldn't be the children. They were my whole life. . . . My whole life was that because I had no life with my husband, the children should make me happy . . . but it never worked out.[4]

Let's imagine a woman like this seeking help from a male therapist (most therapists are male, but a woman therapist might say the same things) at three different points in her life.

As a young woman she is torn because she's in love with a man who wants to get married and settle down. She wants to travel and open herself up to new experiences, but she also feels the pressure to get married. Her therapist "helps" her to see that the development of her warm, supportive nature is more important than her desire for independence. So she gets married and for a time, she is content.

The therapist has offered her a "solution" to her dilemma, but it only works for a couple of years. She feels restless cleaning an empty house and decides to have some kids. Five years later she talks to children all day long, and her husband is practically the only adult she sees. She gets to party with her husband's friends, but has nothing to say to them. She watches soap operas; her husband tells her she's letting herself go. She's tired all the time, often depressed, and can't seem to make herself get out of bed in the morning. At this point, a therapist may "help" her to see that the development of her warm, supportive nature will eliminate boredom and depression and make her more attractive to her husband. He tells her to go on a diet, throw herself into raising her children, and use her creativity to make her house a home.

The therapist has offered her a "solution" to her dilemma, but it only works for a couple of years. Ten years later, the children are seldom at home. She feels self-conscious; she is getting gray hair and has put on a few extra pounds. Her husband is wrapped up in his work, so she has practically nothing to share with him; and she is again cleaning an empty house. She feels neither attractive nor needed.

At this point she may tell a therapist that she is unhappy, but doesn't know why. Her words might be almost exactly the same as those of the woman who told us:

> When I was 38 and my youngest child was entering high school, I began to be very depressed. I went to see a therapist and he told me I felt depressed because no one needed me any more. He said, "There are plenty of children who need a woman like you. If you can't get pregnant, why don't you adopt a child?" So I did. Greg is now 5 years old, starting school, and I feel depressed again. What can I do? I can't keep adopting babies forever.

Now the woman tries to fight the growing feeling that she has never really lived. Her therapist tries to get her to develop her warm, supportive nature by once again making her husband the major focus of her life, taking special care to make herself attractive, appearing interested in her husband's work, and perhaps doing some volunteer work to fill up her free time. That's what she'll look forward to for the rest of her life.

We realize that our description of the therapist's diagnosis sounds simplistic; therapists rarely say these things so directly. But no matter what his/her intentions are, the impact on this woman's life is the same. In accepting psychology's basic assumption that problems are personal and not societal, the therapist has failed to see how this woman's crisis arose quite logically out of her situation, out of her feelings of inadequacy as a woman. The therapist's solutions provided, at best, a patchwork job, and if at any point that husband had disappeared through death or divorce, that patchwork would have dissolved and she would have been left empty and helpless. The therapist's emphasis on her developing her warm, supportive nature meant that she never learned to develop an autonomous, separate identity, much less the skills to support herself in a discriminatory economic market.

An alternative kind of therapy might have shown her how to redefine relationships and responsibilities to her partner and children so that these aspects of her life did not destroy her capacity to develop other parts of herself.

In Ibsen's play *A Doll's House*, Nora and Torvald Helmer confront each other about Nora's decision to stop devoting her entire identity to her husband and children:

Nora: What do you consider my most sacred duties?
Helmer: Do I need to tell you that? Are they not your duties to your husband and your children?
Nora: I have other duties just as sacred.
Helmer: That you have not. What duties could those be?
Nora: Duties to myself.[5]

An alternative kind of therapy, we believe, must begin with the therapist's ability to analyze the *sources* of women's depression and anger. The degree to which much traditional therapy is based on inadequate analysis is evident in the following account, written for us by a student intern about her experience on a psychiatric ward.

One Woman's Problem: Two Interpretations

During the summer of '72, as a student working on a psychiatric ward, I observed and participated in the "therapeutic process." This ward was reputed to be an alternative to the traditional 24-hour psychiatric hospitalization. I found out differently. I found a total absence of any political or social analysis on the part of the staff in interpreting the problems of women on the ward. They overlooked the implications of sex-role socialization and of sex discrimination as being a primary influence on the problems men and women face. "The Word" was that each individual had her own unique problem. An individual solution to her problem was sought or created. Never was any connection made between her problems and the social inequities that were put upon her because she was female, poor, Black, etc.

One woman who came in for therapy is an example: Her situation: *25 years old, white, jobless mother of three young children. She had recently been abandoned by her husband, left with three months' back rent due on a $300-a-month apartment. Her job opportunities were limited since she was married at age 16 and never had the time or need to support herself. Her marriage was unsuccessful. She had been seeing a woman therapist, but she didn't feel the therapy was helping her.*

Because of her money problems she was very upset, nervous, confused. The pressures were becoming unbearable. The welfare people then took her children away for an indefinite period of time because they said she was "inadequate as a mother."

The Staff's Interpretation of Her Problem. After lengthy interviews, it was decided that all her problems has really begun in childhood; her present situation was an extension and only symptomatic of a crisis left unresolved in childhood. Her father had disappeared when she was 5 years old and the staff concluded that, having been denied a father (and thus rendered unable to resolve her Oedipal conflict), her real problem was an inability to relate to men.

In order to calm her down and make her "pliable" for therapy, tranquilizers were prescribed. The staff members thought it best for her to start seeing a male *therapist on a long-term basis. This would enable her to start dealing with her problem of relating to men. Nothing was done about getting her children back or about finding her a way to support herself.*

My Interpretation. After talking with her, it seemed to me her most pressing problem was her lack of self-confidence and her inability to make decisions. As she so openly said, since she was 16, she had always had a man to rely on. Just like most women, her main goal in life had been to catch a man. She had never had time to develop a sense of independence, which comes partly from acquiring practical skills to support herself and her family. Hopefully, if she could develop these skills, she would gain a sense of self-confidence. And with this newly found self-confidence, many of her present pressures would slowly disappear; she could support her family and gain confidence in her ability to make decisions.

The tranquilizers the staff prescribed seemed to be a device to keep her from meeting her problems head-on, and the staff's advice of switching her to a male therapist would only provide one more instance in which she would have to rely on a man, not on herself.

When a woman's problems are so overwhelmingly caused by a society that keeps her helpless and insecure, the kind of therapy she needs is learning ways to overcome these feelings by learning to help herself.

The student intern's experience is a particularly clear example of a general truth about therapy: your therapist's interpretation of the origin and nature of your problems will greatly shape the possible options toward which he or she will direct you. The overtness of direction will vary widely from therapist to therapist because therapists differ considerably on how "directive" they like to be. But your therapist's questions, positive or negative reactions, suggestions, insights, or recommendations will naturally be based on some interpretation of the cause and extent of your problems. The options that follow from that interpretation may involve adjustment, change, or a complex interweaving of the two. One important part you can play in making your therapy successful is to examine your therapist's interpretations critically. Do they really help you understand? Do they ring true? Are they consistent with your notions of who you *can* be and who you *want* to be? Do they open paths for you to experience autonomy, fulfilling human relationships, or a combination of these?

To help you evaluate your therapist and his or her potential affect on your well-being, we will examine the role of authority, stereotyping, masculine norms for female sexuality, and psychological theory in the following chapters. The first crucial aspect of your therapy that you need to examine critically is the dynamics of your relationship with your therapist. What psychological power or authority does he or she exert over you? What is the nature of your trust or admiration of your therapist?

FOOTNOTES

[1]Susan Dworkin Levering, "She Must Be Some Kind of Nut," *Rough Times*, 3, no. 1 (September 1972), 3. First entitled *The Radical Therapist, Rough Times* is now published under the name *State and Mind.*

[2]Ibid.

[3]In Sigmund Freud, "Analysis Terminable and Interminable" (1937), trans. Joan Riviere, in *Therapy and Technique*, Philip Rieff, ed. (New York: Macmillan, 1963), p. 270.

[4]Pauline Bart, "Depression in Middle-Aged Women" in *Woman in Sexist Society*, Vivian Gornick and Barbara K. Moran, eds. (New York: Basic Books, 1971), p. 163.

[5]From Henrik Ibsen, *A Doll's House* (written in 1879), in *Three Plays by Ibsen* (New York: Dell, 1959), p. 157.

The Therapist and Power

Inherent in your therapy situation is an unequal power relationship. Your therapist is usually a man—the Expert—with several degrees after his name. He has the training that is supposed to explain your problems; he is the authority figure who can usually impose his view of things on you. You, on the other hand, are the vulnerable, uncertain person seeking help (if you weren't in such an unconfident state, you probably wouldn't be looking for therapy).

ROLE POWER

Since doctors have very high status in our society, both you and your therapist (like most of us) are likely to trust the word of the Expert over the person in need of help, even if that person is yourself. Unless you or your therapist has consciously struggled against the idea that he is always right

29

because he is your doctor, your therapist is considered the "sane" and "healthy" one while you are somehow "sick" or "maladjusted" or even "crazy." These terms are not always used—a more euphemistic term for you is "patient" —but even unspoken, they may underlie your relationship with your therapist. If your therapist gives you a "diagnosis" (therapists supposedly don't tell you what's "wrong" with you, but it happens all the time, even after only one session), you are expected to accept it, learn from it, and change what he thinks is your "sick" behavior.

If you resist his analysis of your problems, he—with his tremendous aura of authority—will be able to suggest that you don't really want to help yourself, that you are resisting him because you can't face your problem

In *Women and Madness*, Phyllis Chesler recounts the experience of a woman, Sandra, whose challenge to her therapist's authority was turned against her. Sandra was in group therapy with a male psychiatrist in New York City. He was well established, "reputable," with an expensive address, and he ran his group and private sessions very authoritatively, to the point of often dictating with whom his patients should sleep, and what jobs they should take. He insisted that only he could "help" or "save" his patients, and that anyone who stopped therapy left at his or her own risk. Sandra refused to sleep with him when he propositioned her; she told her husband and decided to stop "treatment." Her decision was painfully complicated by his accusations in front of the rest of the group. Chesler quotes Sandra's account of her experience:

> I decided, though, that I owed it to Mark [her husband] to go up with him and confront the group we're all in together. So I got up and there's Doctor X and his two assistants sitting there and I figure, well the cards are stacked against me. . . . Dr. X says, "Well, well, tell us what happened." So I tell the story again and then he proceeds to tell the group how I was provocative to him, how I wore a miniskirt—which I always wear. He made it look as if I were coming up there to seduce him, not to have a session. . . . Then he says I'm using this lie of a proposition to cop out of therapy. He reminded me that I didn't quit a job I once had just because my boss made a pass at me.

... Then all of a sudden we're sitting there and he's starting to say things like: "Sandra, you know how dishonest you are, how dishonest you are with Mark, there are things you haven't told him" [he was referring to a brief affair she'd had], and I started crying, "I'm getting out of here," I mean it was like a kangaroo court . . . and when we left, Mark said to me, "What haven't you told me; what did you do?" He forgot all about what Dr. X did. . . . Everything got twisted.[1]

Since you are likely to be uncertain about yourself and what's making you unhappy, you can easily be convinced by your therapist's assertions that he knows best. A therapist can have an incredible influence on your attitude toward yourself, especially if you have internalized society's belief in the doctor as Expert.

A woman we interviewed told us the story of her therapy:

I went to a therapist who over the months diagnosed me as having "thought disorder." He questioned very closely and critically every-thing I said before pointing out to me all my distortions of the truth. This sounds reasonable, but what it really meant was that he never believed anything I said. It wasn't long before my husband, who was involved in my therapy, didn't believe what I said either ("My dear, you know that's not true; it's your thought disorder again"). And finally I didn't believe what I said or felt anymore. When I tried to write down on paper what I was really feeling, he told me to tear it up and throw it away—it was intellectualizing, part of my craziness. Then my therapist put me on drugs; within a month I had gained 15 pounds. When I told him this gain worried and bothered me (I felt fat—that is, in this society, unattractive) he told me to forget it; it wasn't a problem (Two years later when I saw him by chance, he had lost 100 pounds!)

Whenever I disagreed with the therapist's diagnoses, he would say, "Now Sally, you know you're just distorting again; don't you want to help yourself?" At one point, I tried to commit suicide. While my stomach was being pumped in the hospital, he told me that my at-tempt was not a "real" one. I felt he had taken away the validity of even that desperate act. I finally had the courage to leave this ther-apist, but it was nine months before I had the confidence to speak much to my new therapist or friends. The only protection against having people think I was lying or distorting was not to speak at all. I walked around wrapped in a lonely fear of having no validity, no credibility, no reason for self-confidence. I have slowly regained some of my former self-confidence—though little spontaneity—because of the supportive way my new therapist has listened to how I see my problems.

This power the therapist can have over the "patient's" mind is even greater for the woman in therapy (especially with a male therapist) than for the man. "Healthy" women are expected to be more submissive in their relationships with men or authority than are "healthy" males. If you contradict what your male therapist says to you, he (as a man) may be threatened by your challenge, while he might take such a disagreement from a man as a positive sign of growing self-confidence. If you and your husband or male lover are seeing a male therapist together, you may discover a subtle bond developing between the two men that leaves you out. A double standard of expectations may also emerge.

A woman told us about her couple therapy in these words:

When I was in therapy in a hospital, my husband was asked to join in many of my sessions because the hospital liked family therapy [treat the family situation, not the individual]. At first, I talked a great deal, and the therapist encouraged my husband to speak up, give opinions, etc. Soon the joint sessions became subtly centered on my husband's ideas and feelings, and I became very quiet. Rather than encouraging me to speak, the therapist told me I was sullen because I didn't want to help myself. Instead of listening to me, my husband began to accept what the therapist said about me. I felt I had lost my ally when he would attack me with the therapist's diagnosis. Even after the therapy ended, he would contradict whatever I said about it to friends and explain to them that I said those things because I was mentally ill.

The picture we have drawn of some therapists may seem unreal, as if we see the therapist as a special kind of tyrant. That is not quite the point. Some therapists may in fact be quite explicit about their power, their sense that they are always right, and their belief that their "clients" are sick. But the overwhelming power of the therapist and the person's subservient position is usually not explicit. It is assumed in their roles as "doctor" and "patient." The therapist's self-assurance and authority, and the "client's" tendency to doubt herself are as much a part of their relationship as these factors are in the relationship of a parent to child, a doctor to patients or nurses, and an employer to employees.

One woman told us:

> *When I was about to take my prelim exam for a Ph.D., I went to a psychiatry clinic because I was nervous, distraught, unable to sleep, and suffering from severe stomach upsets. At one point during the therapy, the therapist, after questioning me sharply about why I worked so hard, asked finally, "What makes you think you can pass prelims anyway?"*

This kind of implicit power may be much harder for you to deal with because it can easily go unrecognized by both you and a therapist with good intentions. Some therapists may have struggled not to fall into this authority role, and to view the therapy relationship in terms of two people who are trying to talk through some problems.

What we suggest is that you be aware of this problem in therapy. When you disagree with your therapist, try to watch for his reaction. Keep in mind what we have said, and try to remember that you might be right. A good therapy relationship is probably the one in which there is give and take on both sides—you learn and your therapist learns, too.

SEXUAL POWER

The power the therapist can often have over your mind has all too often extended into a sexual power as well. Women all over the country are beginning to tell stories (and file suits) concerning outright rape by therapists and concerning cases of a more subtle insinuation that an "affair" would be good for the "treatment."

For example, one woman told us:

After a long period of therapy, my therapist told me that he had fallen in love with me. My reaction was impatience—that was his problem and I had my own problems to solve. His response was that I did not know how to give love!

Phyllis Chesler quoted a woman she interviewed who had slept with her therapist:

I know I needed him very, very badly. It was like he was God. . . . He was mistreating me, and I didn't want to admit that because I needed him badly. I loved him. . . . Then he offered me a job as his typist but he wouldn't sleep with me any more. I was so depressed and upset and I wanted some help and called up, hysterical, "Please talk to me on the phone," and he said, "I can't talk to you now, I'll call you back." And he never called back. I felt deserted and all alone and usually when I talk about this with my shrink [now] I'm just in tears.[2]

There is even a whole school of therapy that insists on sex between therapists (overwhelmingly male) and their "patients" (overwhelmingly female). "Touch therapy" and "the love treatment" are terms often associated with the therapy that sex between you and your therapist is a useful part of a "cure."

Chesler quoted Sheila, a woman she interviewed:

I got stoned on grass because I was so scared. . . . I was up for having an affair, but this didn't feel like an affair. . . . He told me I was blocked, that there were things I had to work out with my father and that maybe we could solve it on a non-verbal level if I would just trust him . . . and that I was going to have to trust him. . . . So maybe he's bizarre and unattractive—I didn't feel too straight myself. . . . Oh, God. Then he got up, dropped his pants, said, "Take your pants down," or something really insensitive, unsensual and he just got on top of me. He came, I didn't come. And then I said, "I'd like to get on top of you." And then he told me that that was my problem, that I wanted to be in control. . . .[3]

Nancy Caughran wrote of a similar experience:

> I had been to therapy with Phineas for two and a half years when he offered to have an affair with me ... at a time when I was feeling particularly depressed and confused about leaving graduate school and other things. Phineas, one day, gave me the choice of continuing therapy with him or "making it" together. I was struck numb and unable to reply with much of anything. He tried to make it sound inviting, laughingly adding something about keeping sado-masochistic pleasures within the confines of the bedroom. When I walked out of his office, I was somewhat elated, thinking, "Wow! He knows how messed up I am and still he's attracted to me!" But that feeling of elation was based on the old bullshit of "You're OK if you get approval from a man!" And approval meant that I was attractive to him in some way.
>
> ... This being my first experience in therapy, I was quite vulnerable —as most patients are. Using this vulnerability, he had subtly and not so subtly encouraged me to depend on him and invest him with a great deal of power. In this context, my sexual thoughts and fantasies were probed. He asked me often about my sexual feelings for him, and if I said that I didn't think I had any, it was suggested that I was repressing them. As a result, I was led to feel that not spending time fantasizing about being with him in bed indicated something was wrong with me. ...
>
> The next two months were perhaps the worst I'd ever gone through. I really can't describe the agony. I felt totally powerless—there seemed nothing I could do. *After all, he was the therapist, with all the letters after his name; I was merely the patient.* Who would believe *me?*[4]

Caughran went on to describe how she escaped her situation and feelings of powerlessness. She attended a workshop on psychiatry and rape at a women's conference. Learning to see her experience as a reflection of a wide-scale social problem instead of her own "craziness," she went with some of the women from the conference to confront Phineas at one of the group sessions. The result for her was new strength and self-respect: she felt "really pleased that I did what I did. ... Perhaps the best effect for me was to clarify that Phineas no longer has power over me. I see him very differently now.

He's no longer god and certainly not powerful. But, he is very dangerous, and I feel badly that he, and others like him, can continue to abuse this very one-sided power relationship for their own ends."[5]

If you are in therapy because you feel enormously vulnerable and inadequate, you may easily be sucked into a therapist's need to exercise some form of power over his women patients. The first step in escaping such "one-sided power" relationships is evaluating your therapist's actions and your feelings in the wider context of power relations between men and women in general.

THE POWER OF AUTHORITY

A therapist's power does not have to be expressed in overtly sexual ways for its psychological impact to be shattering. We include here an extended account a woman wrote for us on how the therapist's authority can destroy confidence, indeed one's very identity.

Case Study: The Power to Destroy

When my husband very suddenly left me and went to live with a close friend of mine, I was totally wiped out by what I experienced as a complete rejection of me as a person and especially as a woman. My life loomed before me as a total blank. I sat for hours staring at the wall. It was a leap of faith that kept me taking the pill every morning. I was a student at the time, and at the first exam, I froze and couldn't write. My sense of failure as a wife spread to everything I did. I was seeing a therapist (a young guy—wore his McCarthy button all the time) because I didn't know what else to do—I had no close friends and couldn't burden my acquaintances with so much pain. I clung to each week's session as my only straw because who else could I talk to just about myself? Week after week the therapist would lead me to talk about all the things I did—I played tournament tennis, I was a teacher, a graduate student, a one-time musician, etc. Once I told him I had played basketball with my husband and his friend; I had astounded them by shooting seventeen free throws without a miss; I was stopped by the friend suddenly blocking my eighteenth try (he sprained his finger!). The therapist's response was, "Why are you telling me this: Why do you have to create such myths about yourself?"

I know now why I told him this story—I was so crushed and unconfident that I clung to any symbol of success or of potential. And in the context of his approach, I was somewhat desperately trying to convince him, *as well as myself, that there was some reason to respect me. He had been saying to me that sometimes it's best to break down everything and start at rock bottom (I think he even used the words "tear down" and "destroy"). And tear me down he had been systematically doing. Each thing I had told him I thought I had been doing well (but now I wasn't sure anymore), he broke down and showed me how it was nothing.*

I agreed with him. I was nothing. I had no brains, no ability as an athlete or competitor, no musical talent, no potential as a teacher, no friends. I became more and more depressed, but I never considered quitting or changing therapists. My father was nearly frantic over the phone to get me to quit. The man I had tentatively begun to see told me the therapist was threatened by me and I had lost all perspective on my marriage—my husband was the schmuck, not me. But I didn't listen to them. Deep down, I knew the therapist was right— he must be because for years I had had regular depressions centering on inner conviction of failure and now my husband had left me because of it.

By the seventh week of therapy, my confidence about everything I had done outside my marriage was completely destroyed. I was at rock bottom and totally passive—anything he said must be true. Then he said it was time to talk about my marriage—how could I have thought it was a happy marriage for at least five years? He had seen me "crucify my husband" in the one joint session my husband had agreed to attend. I was a woman with too many drives and too many myths about myself. My husband couldn't take living with me. I had destroyed his confidence, etc., etc., etc. I could see the direction my therapist was heading—my biggest failure was as a wife and woman. I was a castrator. For the first time in weeks, there were stirrings inside me that he must be wrong. Years ago, I had read The Feminine Mystique. *Men who called women "castrating bitches" had a problem. I had* not *been that way to my husband—I knew that even then I had been* too *dependent; I had centered my life too much on him and he had become uncomfortable with the pressure. (As for the joint therapy session, I did at that time feel guilty about speaking so forcefully about my husband. Now I can see that that session was the* only *time I was able to express my anger or hurt to my husband. Alone with him, I was understanding, always blaming myself and trying to get him to talk about his feelings. Women tend to have a problem expressing anger toward a man—a good therapist would have encouraged me to get those violent, furious feelings out in the open.) I began to disagree a little bit with the therapist—"No. I don't think it was quite like that." "I don't think so"—all very tentative. But I still had not thought of changing therapists or quitting. My later slow, painful growth toward strength and confidence owes a great deal to his angry response to my disagreement because it pushed me to quit. His face got red. I have this image of him huffing and puffing. He told me I couldn't disagree with him like that—he didn't use any fancy terms like "repression" or "projection." He just said straight out that I couldn't oppose him like that. And next week I would have to lie down on the couch, where it would be much harder to disagree. I would be more receptive to what he had to say. Then we could make progress. Thank God he was so blatant. If he had been more indirect, I would never have quit.*

I sometimes ask myself why I was such a sucker for his line. I had believed, consciously at least, that women should be independent. I had never pictured a life revolving around children and husband as right for me. But I actually had helped that therapist tear me to pieces limb by limb. Does this prove that women are after all masochistic?

There was no woman's movement at the time to help me think through these issues. But I now see how this therapist's indirectly expressed attitudes toward me and women and his openly destructive method blended in with and intensified the kinds of insecurities I felt and so many other women feel as a result of growing up female in this country. The fear of failure as a wife: a woman is worthless if she can't hold her man; a fear of failure in the man's world: I had rejected the traditional woman's role, but I was wracked by insecurity that I couldn't make it in the world of achievement (a feeling reinforced by attitudes and discrimination on the outside—e.g., woman athletes are not real athletes; no money for women's sports). Fear of openly admitting my successes—women should not shine outside the home and certainly shouldn't outshine their husbands. In so many ways, I was caught in a classic woman's bind. All the therapist did was to tie the knots tighter. The strength to unwind the strangling ropes could have come, I suppose, from a therapist who fostered self-confidence and independence, but I was in no shape to look for another therapist on the rebound from the first experience. As it was, I escaped first of all by talking to other people, especially women, looking at the troubles of other couples, reading about women, and finally developing the awareness that what I had experienced was part of a larger pattern. But understanding and friendships were not enough by them-

selves. I still had to face those inner fears and depressions "all by myself" (the childhood refrain that are my daughter's favorite words). Alone.

THE POWER OF PSYCHOLOGICAL THEORY AND TERMINOLOGY

The development of a potentially destructive power relationship in therapy can originate not only in your therapist's needs but also in some of the standard "tools of the trade"—that is, psychological theory and terminology. The concept of "defense mechanisms" is one such common "tool"—one you should evaluate carefully.

"Defense Mechanisms": The Power to Twist Your Words

Freud was the first psychologist to label some of the things we say and do as "defense mechanisms." Defense mechanisms are said to occur when buried feelings, desires, or ideas are diverted into something different. Although few therapists today call themselves "Freudian," his terminology for "defense mechanisms"—repression, reaction formation, projection, sublimation, fixation, regression—is still widely used to explain people's problems and especially people's so-called refusal to recognize their problems.

These "defense mechanisms" may indeed represent a brilliant insight on Freud's part. All of us may repress things we don't want to face, or "project" our own feelings onto others, or "regress" into childish behavior, or "sublimate" some desire into acceptable action. These concepts, when used very carefully and with great restraint on the part of your therapist, may illuminate some hidden aspect of your difficulties. But as a tool in the analysis of your problems, the concept of "defense mechanisms" *can be very dangerous and destructive* to you. With this terminology, the therapist can always invalidate what *you* say and claim that what *he* or *she* says is correct. If "defense mechanisms" are used this way, you can never come out ahead—any statement you make can be twisted into evidence for your therapist's ideas about your state of emotional health.

Even with the kindest intentions, his or her preconceptions about you personally or about women in general always have the arsenal of defense-mechanism terminology to justify his/her words as "scientific": the therapist is right and you are just "resisting," "projecting," "sublimating," or whatever. This power that the therapist holds over you can make you question any genuine feelings you have. The danger for you is that you can so easily be caught in a bind, especially if you are very unhappy and unsure of yourself to begin with. Either you must accept your therapist's interpretation or the whole experience becomes frustrating, sometimes terrifying, especially as you try to convince your therapist that your own thoughts are valid and that "defense mechanisms" may not be operating.

If your therapist uses these terms with you, you may easily feel intimidated by their scientific tone. Understanding what they mean will help demystify them and break down their power to intimidate. If your therapist avoids using technical terminology, he or she may still use the *concepts* in analysis of your problems. In this case, you will need to be familiar with these concepts.[6] Here, then, are some concrete definitions and examples of these concepts:

Repression. When your therapist says you are "repressing," this means he/she thinks you are forcing an anxious, distressing, or threatening thought out of your mind. For example, if a woman tells her therapist she enjoys being with women more often than with men, he may counter with the observation that she's repressing a memory of a bad experience she once had with a man, a father perhaps. He may ask her to dig up some childhood experience to prove his label. His assumption may be that it is "abnormal" to enjoy being with women more than men; and he can use the terminology of defense mechanisms to obscure his personal bias.

Reaction Formation. To most therapists this means that if your needs or drives appear threatening to you, they may be converted into what seem to be their opposites. Suppose, for example, a woman tells her therapist that she sees herself as a devoted wife and mother but, for some unknown reason, she has recently felt very anxious when she's been cooped up in the house all day doing chores. Her therapist may tell her that what's really operating is a strong emotional response of hatred for her husband and children. According to the therapist, this hatred, being unacceptable, has been converted into an overly loving devotion.

Florence Rush wrote about how a therapist can use the concept of reaction formation in a destructive way:

> One who protects herself from her own drives and converts them into the opposite is using the defense mechanism of *reaction formation.* The housewife who has repressed an infantile wish to play with her feces can [according to some therapists] become compulsively clean, or the woman who hates her husband and children can become an overly devoted wife and mother.[7]

Projection. This means that someone, some situation (even your therapist) is making you so anxious that the only way of dealing with the difficulty is by evading personal responsibility for your actions and transferring that responsibility to something or someone else. Say, for example, that a woman believes her boss is discriminating against her because she's a woman. As a result, she is very frustrated and begins to hate her boss, and other men at work. A therapist may explain this by saying she really hates herself because she can't function as well as she should and needs to blame someone else for her failure.

Sublimation. Unlike the other "defense mechanisms," this one is good for you (supposedly). Sublimation means that instead of repressing your drives, you express them in socially acceptable ways. For example, if a woman expresses great delight when she discovers she is pregnant, the therapist may attribute this delight to her successful and socially acceptable fulfillment of her long-term underlying basic desire to have a penis.

Again quoting from Rush's critique of destructive use of defense-mechanism terminology:

> Sublimation is also a defense mechanism but [is seen as] a good and healthy one. The sublimation of unconscious drives results not in the repression of energy, but its conversion into socially acceptable behavior. The man with an overpowering urge toward voyeurism can become a psychiatrist and satisfy his curiosity by looking at and helping people at the same time and the woman who wants a penis can have a baby instead and be a mother.[8]

Regression. Regression means that you are going back to an earlier stage of development. Say a housewife is bored with her housework and feels the need to get out of the house to meet her friends for lunch and a movie. A therapist might conclude she is trying to recapture the freedom of her premarital days. The assumption here is that a woman can or should feel content in the home; if she is not, then she must be "regressing" instead of responding to a genuine dissatisfaction and a *real* problem in her situation.

Fixation. This means remaining at a certain stage of development instead of progressing to a subsequent stage. Suppose a woman gets a job in a male-dominated field and she constantly finds herself in conflict with her employers and colleagues. The therapist may interpret her rebellion as fixation: during the Oedipal phase of psycho-sexual development (when, according to Freud, girls compete in fantasy with their mothers for the sexual love of their fathers), she became angry with her father for rejecting her. In her adult life, the therapist may explain, she is fixated at this stage of angry rebellion against men. The therapist, using the concept of fixation, might not see alternative explanations of anger—that the woman is justifiably angry with the discriminatory treatment she receives from some men at work.

The danger of using these Freudian interpretations is that they are part of a closed system. This means that no matter how hard you deny that these mechanisms are *not* operating, the therapist can potentially argue that you're unconsciously making use of them, that you're unaware of the forces operating within yourself. In this closed system, the therapist is *never* wrong and your own feelings are never valid. If your therapist explains your problems by referring to these terms or concepts, or writes them in your file, or uses them with other therapists, remember how easily they can be used to prove you wrong. Remember also how subtly they point the finger of blame to something buried inside you and away from some genuine problem in your situation, something *external* to you.

Rush wrote about herself when she was a mother with a young child who rarely slept at night and constantly demanded her attention:

> I dreamt that I was pursued by a man dressed in black. He was a policeman carrying a club and I was very anxious to escape him. I became very tired and almost ready to allow my pursuer to catch me when there appeared a smaller figure also in black carrying a club who filled me with such terror that I made a last desperate effort to run. In a panic I awoke to the sound of Bobby's voice in my ear babbling, "Mommy get up and play choo choo train with me."
>
> Sensing that this was an important dream, I free associated, came up with a few clues of my own and with the help of Dr. Jones a breakthrough was made and I gained an insight: The two figures pursuing me were my husband and son. They appeared to me as policemen because I found them threatening and in black cloaks because I feared them at night. The clubs were of course the penis and I was running from the symbol of male aggression, manhood, and the masculinity of my husband and son. I had previously explained to Dr. Jones that I had often rejected my husband's sexual advances because I was exhausted from lack of sleep. The dream revealed that I rejected my

husband's sexual advances, not from exhaustion, but from underlying hostility and fear of men.[9]

If you doubt the validity of your therapist's analysis, don't just dismiss that doubt; explore it, think critically about what the therapist has said, and *express* your doubts. Be suspicious if your therapist contradicts everything you say and refers to your "defense mechanisms." Ask yourself if the therapist's explanations contain any assumptions about women, as those of Dr. Jones did. Some "defense mechanisms" may be operating, but it is just as likely they are not. See if you can think of any other explanations to explain your feelings—especially explanations that take into account the *real* difficulties in your situation. Don't allow your therapist to use these terms to twist all your words into something that you believe is foreign and untrue to your feelings. The result of unquestioning acceptance of what a therapist says might be the destruction of your self-confidence and the loss of a chance for independence and trust in yourself.

The ways in which technical psychological terminology and concepts can gradually undermine your trust in your own perceptions is demonstrated forcefully by another extended account of an experience in therapy. We quote directly from Nicole Anthony's widely reprinted "Open Letter to Psychiatrists."[10]

Case Study: Open Letter to Psychiatrists

A few years ago I went to see a well-known psychiatrist in San Francisco. I was very unhappy in my role as mother-housewife—supportive woman behind the man. He told me that I needed intensive therapy and began to see me several times a week privately and once a week in one of his "groups." He suggested that after therapy, I would be happy to stay at home and be a "woman," happy to serve my husband and children.

The psychiatric profession is built on the slavery of women. Oppressive definitions of woman underlie all of its theory and most of its practice. When a woman protests the slave-servant role she is labeled emotionally ill.

At the beginning of each hour the good doctor would greet me with a hug and a pat on the rear. The hug, I believed, was meant to be warm, but the pat felt strangely inexplicable. During the hour he would pull his chair right beside mine; he believed in "close" interaction with his patients. Sometimes he leaned over and placed his hand on my stomach or thigh with an outright grin of possession. I would squirm and put my head down in discomfort, and if feeling particularly brave, I would say "But that's not appropriate," whereupon he would leer and answer, "But why not? Are you afraid I can't control myself?" With a subtle twist of words he implied that my response to his aggression was a PROJECTION of my own secret wishes to "sleep with my father." I wasn't afraid that he couldn't control himself; obviously he couldn't control himself. I was afraid to admit that he really was leering, afraid he would tell me I was distorting, projecting, fantasizing and INSANE. And what can you do when your psychiatrist tells you you're crazy and everyone says that psychiatrists are the ones to judge your emotional health?

When women talk about the vicious and ugly things that men feel free to do to them the psychiatrists mumble jumble about projections and who would believe a woman. When women get raped on the streets psychiatrists say that they wanted to be raped.

After awhile my therapy got sticky. The good doctor carefully explained how I had a super-thin membrane separating my conscious and unconscious thoughts, likening me to a borderline schizophrenic. Since my thin membrane made me think things were real when they weren't, my perceptions of reality must be suspect. Obviously any perceptions I had about him that weren't favorable could be thrown out as products of sickness.

When women step out of line and refuse to submit, psychiatrists quickly apply some meaningless "descriptive" label to their behavior and often send them to punitive institutions, all in the name of mental health.

Finally, my therapist began forgetting and coming late to appointments. One hour late, he whizzed into his waiting room in tennis clothes at our last meeting. I had been nervously thumbing through back issues of the New Yorker, worrying about my borderline membrane that perceived this therapeutic situation as very peculiar. I was scared and hurt. I told him I thought his behavior strange, and he mumbled about my distortions and how therapists were also human. That evening I called my uncle, who is a psychiatrist in another city. I didn't tell him much, only that I felt something was wrong in my therapy, that my therapist thought I was projecting, that I certainly wanted to stick with him and "work it out" if that was the case, but if in fact he was having some "counter-transference" problem I wanted a quick out and a new doctor. My psychiatrist uncle said I should ask for a consultation, a very common and legitimate thing to do which would clear the matter up. He was kind and sympathetic, and I think confused about the state of his crazy niece. I telephoned my therapist and asked for a consultation with a reputable psychoanalyst from the San Francisco Psychoanalytic Institute. My therapist got very angry. No, he would not agree to a consultation because of my crazy projections and distortions, and furthermore, he didn't like the idea of a patient telling him "how to conduct his medical practice," and a patient had no right to bring others in to meddle in his BUSINESS. Therapy was terminated.

Shaking about my membrane, and terrified of the hate which I had felt from my ex-therapist, I went to see the psychoanalyst from the Institute. It took a long time to undo the damage, to reassure myself that yes, my perceptions were right on, no, I wasn't suffering from membrane problems. My new therapist sat by, listening and making it clear that he didn't think I was crazy at all. He didn't pat my stomach and thigh and ask why I didn't dig it.

Not all psychiatrists systematically try to destroy their female patients.

My ex-therapist is still in practice. Occasionally, I meet other women who were in therapy with him, and each describes a similar experience; the pats, the squeezes, the leers, the subtle implications and accusations of insanity. We think we should sue him for malpractice but we are afraid because he knows all the intimate details of our lives that we don't want made public for the sake of our families as well as ourselves. I could cite three dozen other such doctors.

Psychiatrists can continue to exploit and brutalize women with complete impunity, protected by the nature of their work from any legal actions that might limit the damage done. We are angry and soon there will be enough of us to move against those doing evil in the name of therapy. Psychiatrists, listen now.

We have all heard the familiar phrases, "pull yourself up by the bootstraps, pull yourself together, have some self-respect and others will treat you with respect, stop oppressing yourself and others will stop oppressing you." The psychiatrists tell us about "internalization," implying that we internalize the norms, the contempt held for us by those in power, and act as our own prison guards. It's a lie. When we step out of line, when we act with strength and self-love we are pun-

ished. Sometimes the punishment is clear, like getting fired when we refuse to serve the boss coffee with a sweet feminine smile, or getting beat up when we "talk back" to our husbands. More often the punishment is subtle and takes place in a series of warning gestures that we call gestures of dominance. They carry with them a threat of violence should they fail to do the job. They are subtle and often barely perceptible.

Women are especially sensitive to gestures. Their survival has depended on correctly assessing the moods of their masters and that mood is communicated through gestures.

When a dominant chimpanzee wants to sit in a place occupied by a less dominant chimp, he gives a gesture of dominance, maybe a sound and a direct stare, and the lower-ranking chimp responds with a gesture of submission, often some variation of "presenting," and quickly moves over to make room for the boss. If he or she fails to submit, the dominant chimp resorts to violence.

Chorus girls turn their asses to the male audience: present, present. My therapist pats my ass: present, present.

Sometimes, in the middle of a heated discussion with a man, a strong woman finds herself acting chimp-like. I'm oppressing myself, she thinks, why do I act like a schmuck, I don't need to act like this, the psychiatrist says I oppress myself, I internalize, etc.

If we filmed the scene we would see that what really happened was that he gave a gesture of dominance and she submitted in fear.

There's no need to submit, the psychiatrists say. Another lie. If a woman refuses to respond to the gestures of dominance she is frequently physically attacked. A wife needs only to be hit by a husband larger and heavier than she. Thereafter the most fleeting subliminal gesture will serve to remind her of the costs of rebellion.

The moments of "internalization" are really the moments when we respond to gestures of dominance. They are not inside of our heads.

The chimpanzee is not born knowing the gestures of his group. Monkeys raised in isolation from their peer group do not learn the appropriate gestures of social communication and grow up unable to have normal social and sexual relationships. Curled up in a corner, they rock and exhibit other stereotypic behaviors that remind one of autistic children. They cannot communicate with their fellow monkeys.

The gestures of social communication are not instinctive. They are learned in early childhood and reinforced throughout life.

There is nothing "natural" about the condition of women. It has been, and remains, in the material interest of men to have women working for them. Recent research makes it increasingly clear that all behavior is learned; even the behavior of the autonomic nervous system is subject to learning, and certainly the functioning of the endocrine system is greatly affected by learning. Aggression is a learned response to external events. Passivity is a learned response to events.

They teach us to respond to aggression directed against us with passivity; if we forget they remind us with gestures of dominance; if we still don't remember, they resort to violence. And then they talk about the masochistic tendencies of women as if magical "instinctive" forces were at work.

By the time we get to psychiatrist, we know all about "internalizations, distortions, projections, acting out, masochistic tendencies" with which they claim we are afflicted but in fact which are inflicted upon us. The job of the psychiatrist has been to help us adjust to our oppression by once and for all laying the blame completely on our manipulated and oppressed "psyches." In fact our psyches have nothing to do with what's happening.

Psychiatrists listen: Throw out your old theories which are based on the oppression of women. Listen to your women patients. They will teach you what's really happening.

Psychiatrists listen: We demand reparation for all the damage done. The years of pain, the millions of dollars, the endless list of deaths.

Psychiatrists listen: We demand that you free all political prisoners locked away in your special corrective prisons. Set our sisters free.

FILES AND CONFIDENTIALITY: THE POWER TO INFLUENCE YOUR REPUTATION

The potential hazards of a destructive power relationship developing in therapy are focused mainly in a psychological dimension. Instead of expanding your horizons, therapy can reduce them by eroding confidence and forcing you into a prescribed feminine role. On a much more practical level, however, your therapist also has the power to reveal information about you and the state of your "mental health" that can seriously affect other people's perceptions of you. Most people who go into therapy are feeling so overwhelmed by their psychological problems that they give no thought to the more mundane matters of therapy.

Does your therapist take notes or tape your sessions? Does someone keep a file on you with notes, reports, test scores, and so forth? Who has access to these files? Will your therapist speak with your family, friends, employers, potential employers, (etc.) about your problems without telling you? If the nature of your problem is kept confidential, what about the simple fact that you are in therapy? These are questions we introduce not to induce paranoia, but to make you aware of potential risks.

There is no single answer to these questions that will hold true in general. Therapists and institutions that offer therapy have different stated policies about what they do with all the information, test scores, reports, and "diagnoses" they collect about patients. Some keep very scanty files; others maintain more complete records. Some keep all files under lock and key, with numbers instead of names, and others keep their files with a receptionist. Some insist that they *never* give out any information about a person in therapy, and others openly admit that they pass along information from your file or even the simple fact that you're in therapy.

We advise you to ask about your therapist's policies, but keep in mind that a stated policy is not necessarily an accurate reflection of what really happens. There is no point in your seeing a therapist if you continually feel you must censor what you say for fear of information leaks. But you should be aware that such leaks are a possibility. Try to evaluate what some of the consequences might be if information about your therapy became available to certain people.

The issue of confidentiality is one that affects men as well as women in therapy. As common as therapy is in this country, there is still considerable lack of confidence in people who are labeled "mentally ill." This issue, however, is of special importance for women because of the overlap in common stereotypes of women and mental illness. A widespread prejudice against women is the belief that women are naturally more emotional and flighty, less stable and reliable, than men.

These prejudices parallel the images of people in therapy and thus doubly intensify the frequent distrust in women's capacity to assume responsibility and independence.

The impact of such doubt can be especially serious for women in the job market. Particularly if a woman has a job or is applying for a job in a male-dominated area, she has to be better qualified and perform better than her male counterpart. In order to prove she's not a "flighty female," she has to be twice as stable as any man. In order to prove she's not "scatterbrained," she has to be twice as organized as any man. Her weaknesses are noticed more quickly and are often related to the fact that she is a woman. Consequently, a report stating that a woman is or has been in therapy can feed all the suspicions people around her might like to believe. The report wouldn't even have to say what her problem was—their fantasies would fill in what the report left out. And the job or promotion might go to an "equally competent" male.

Who in particular might want to find out about your therapy? If you are a student, deans and faculty might make your therapy (the fact of therapy more than the diagnoses of therapy) a part of your regular file. For example, a young woman told us:

> *I went to a woman's college. In the position as a student leader, I found out that the Dean of Women knew which women were seeing a therapist. Nothing was a secret.*

If you think you will ever need a reference or letter of recommendation, you should be aware that people can easily be influenced in their evaluation of your future performance by the knowledge that you are in therapy. In particular, a young person who has tried to commit suicide or who has been hospitalized may be considered a poor risk for professional schools and all kinds of employment for which emotional stability is desirable. Where people know the nature of your problems, the risk can be even greater.

For example, Graham Blaine described the fate of one student's application:

> A student who has had a psychotic episode, is now in treatment four times a week with an outside therapist, and has been twice hospitalized for acute alcoholism, presents a form to be filled out as part of his application for law school. One question is, "Has this student been treated for an emotional illness? If so, when, by whom, for how long and what was the diagnosis?" The form is to be returned to the director of admissions.
>
> A letter is sent stating that we do not supply medical or psychological information to admission committees but are willing to write to the medical service at the school about students. A fairly detailed report is sent to a physician connected with the law shool, if it is requested, with the suggestion that the medical director make a general recommendation to the admission committee based on our report.[11]

If you are applying for a government job, particularly one in which you would deal with "sensitive" or "classified" material, your psychiatric background might be investigated. If you happen to be a lesbian and have been in therapy for any sort of problem, your therapist might be asked questions about your sexual preference. The FBI and police may pressure your therapist or even a receptionist for any information about your therapy that they can get. Offices may not routinely be burglarized for information, but governmental agencies regularly seek information about people in therapy for a variety of purposes.

Again, from Blaine:

> An FBI agent calls to discuss a former patient and has a signed release from the student who is now applying for a responsible government position. While in college this boy had sought help for homosexual activity in high school and once in college. The agent needs the answers to three specific questions. Did this man drink too much? Did he indicate that he was in any way disloyal to this country? Did he engage in homosexual practices? This is a difficult problem—one involving loyalty to patient and to country.[12]

Your therapist may feel caught in a moral dilemma, torn between the demands of confidentiality and the needs of the community as he or she perceives them. One writer warns:

> It is vitally important that nothing a student says to a college psychiatrist in confidence be divulged to anyone without the patient's permission. Of course if a patient is overtly psychotic, suicidal or homicidal, the safety of the community must take precedence over maintaining confidence.[13]

It is not only jobs, however, that can be at stake in the confidentiality issue. Therapists can also choose to involve your family in the therapy—without your permission or knowledge. Here is what one student had to say about this:

> *I was having lost of problems with my parents being overprotective. One day my therapist told me that he had called my parents, talked to them about me, and asked them to come up to school. The result was predictable—my parents became twice as protective as before.*

This kind of experience is probably more likely to happen with young people because the therapist can so easily become a sort of substitute parent making decisions for the child-patient. But it can occur with great complications for women of all ages. We are not opposed to "family therapy," but we do believe you should be involved in any decision about extending the therapy to other people.

So what should you do about confidentiality? Just as there is no universal policy on the part of therapists and institutions, there is no simple answer that can serve the needs of all people in therapy. At the very least, find out what your therapist's policy is. If you are concerned about confidentiality, speak frankly with your therapist about the subject. The very fact that you talk about it may prevent him or her from making casual revelations or from not consulting you first. If you are a student, you should look carefully at the possible consequences of revealing information about your therapy to deans (many students tell deans about personal problems and therapy in order to get "incompletes" for courses, drop courses, etc.; this information regularly goes into student files). If you want to talk about any illegal activities with your therapist, you need to be especially aware of the risks of information leaks.

Our advice that you question your therapist closely about confidentiality brings into sharp relief the difficult issue of the therapist's potential power—and potential misuse of power. We have looked at various kinds of power in this chapter—psychological power, "scientific" power, role power, the power of words, and terms used by the therapist, sexual power, and the power to influence others' views of you. But these dangerous powers are all part of the general paradoxical nature of therapy. Even at its best, therapy necessarily involves contradictions. At the very time you are feeling most vulnerable and insecure, you need to develop trust in your reactions so that you can evaluate whether your therapist is destructive or constructive for you. That is, when you most want "expert" advice, you need to guard against seeing your therapist as "the Expert." And conversely, when your therapist does in fact have more experience than you, he or she needs to develop the respect and warmth for you that provides a good climate for your growth. At the very time you need to develop greater strength and independence, your therapy involves you in a dependent relationship. In order for therapy to work for you, trust in and open communication with your therapist is absolutely necessary. But to protect yourself from being hurt by a destructive therapist, you must be willing to question and evaluate.

Do these contradictions make good therapy impossible? We don't think so. And the more readily your therapist understands these paradoxes, the more likely he or she will be able to create an atmosphere that can promote your growth.

FOOTNOTES

[1]Phyllis Chesler, *Women and Madness* (New York: Doubleday, 1972), pp. 150-51. Excerpts from *Women and Madness* by Phyllis Chesler. Copyright © 1972 by Phyllis Chesler. Reprinted by permission of Doubleday & Company, Inc. and Penguin Books Ltd.

[2]Ibid., p. 146.

[3]Ibid., pp. 147–48.

[4]Nancy Caughran, "Psychiatry as Rip-Off," in *Radical Psychology*, Phil M. Brown, ed. (New York: Harper & Row, Publishers, Inc., 1973), pp. 490–92.

[5]Ibid., p. 496.

[6]We are indebted to Florence Rush, whose perceptive article "Who's Afraid of Margaret Ribble?", critical of traditional psychiatry, first directed our attention to the importance of the intimidating nature of defense mechanism terminology. See the special issue on women and psychology, *Rough Times*, 3, no. 1 (September 1972), 6–9. *Rough Times* was formerly published under the name *Radical Therapist*; it is now called *State and Mind*.

[7]Ibid., p. 7.

[8]Ibid.

[9]Ibid., p. 10.

[10]By Nicole Anthony, published in *Radical Therapist*, 1, no. 3 (August 1970). © Reprinted from the *Radical Therapist*.

[11]Graham Blaine, "Divided Loyalties: The College Therapist's Responsibility to the Student, the University and the Parents," *American Journal of Orthopsychiatry*, 34, no. 3 (April 1964), 483. See also Thomas Szasz's discussion of Blaine's material in his "The Psychiatrist: A Policeman in the Schools" in *This Book is About Schools*, Satu Repo, ed. (New York: Random House, 1970).

[12]Ibid., p. 484.

[13]Dana L. Farnsworth, "Concepts of Educational Psychiatry," *Journal of the American Medical Association*, 181, no. 10 (September 1962), 818; also cited in Szasz, "The Psychiatrist: A Policeman in the Schools."

The Therapist, Gender Identity, and Sex Roles

A girl cannot grow into womanhood in American society without general cultural attitudes about the nature and role of women having some sort of profound influence on her identity. Each woman reacts to these normative values with her own unique mixture of acceptance and rebellion. But whatever the individual problems she might bring to therapy, they will almost inevitably intersect in some way with how she has responded to this socialization process. Consequently, in this chapter we will explore how cultural ideas of what is "normal" and desirable for women's psychology and lifestyle enter into therapy. This will include some discussion of how therapy can usefully examine the impact of a woman's childhood on her adult identity; what traditional and nontraditional therapy have had to say about a "healthy" gender identity for women; and what the prejudice against homosexuality as "sick" has meant for lesbians in therapy. These discussions are meant to be a broad guideline to help you evaluate how well your identity and role as a woman is understood and dealt with in your therapy.

CHILDHOOD SOCIALIZATION

A woman who read an early draft of this book told us:

> *I think your putdown of therapists who ask questions about your parents and childhood is too superficial. It can be very relevant to talk about your past. I was sort of chubby as a teenager and my father weighed me in every Sunday in front of the family. It was humiliating for me, and lots of my present insecurities about my body and my worth as a person go back to those weekly weigh-ins.*

Our childhood *is* important to who we are now, what problems we find ourselves tangled in, and the strength or insecurity with which we face them. Whatever the impact of inherited qualities and structures, whatever the particular pressures of the immediate situation, we are at least partially the result of a long process of socialization. At the present moment, we all live in a social context that defines us—our job or lack of one, our lovers, husbands, children, parents, friends, religion, group identity, government, economy, etc. And when we were little, we were also part of a social context that helped to shape the future adult. Our parents or immediate extended family may have constituted the single most important agent of socialization—for good or bad, or most likely, a mixture of both.

And so, if it is done within the perspective of this socialization, talking with your therapist about your mother, father, brothers and sisters, and your particularly vivid childhood experiences, can be very relevant. Fragments of memories, dreams involving your family, buried feelings about your past can be helpful gold mines, as Freud says—*but not* if they are analyzed in a "Freudian" way. When your childhood memories are examined for what they can reveal about the origins of your feelings about yourself as a woman and your ability to handle the difficulties women face, then your past *can* help illuminate your present. Your mother, or another woman (or women) close to you as a child, was probably your most important role model—the person you looked up to, unconsciously or consciously imitated, or rebelled against as you gradually developed by whatever route you took from girlhood to womanhood. Your father, or other men near you, probably formed your earliest ideas about what men are like or how they treat women. Your feelings about your parents and their influence on you may be crucial determinants of the way you deal in the present with the restrictions you face as a woman.

Just to set you thinking about your own childhood, here are some of the relevant questions about childhood socialization that you might want to explore with your therapist: Were your parents disappointed not to have a son, in spite of their love for you? Did their treatment of you change when you got a brother? Would they have brought you up differently if you had had a brother? Did they give you dolls, pretty dresses, and sewing kits or baseball gloves, microscopes, and trucks? Or both? Did they reinforce "tough" or "coy," "delicate" behavior? (You might be able to answer this by watching your parents with younger sisters or with your own children.) Did the men in your family and/or visitors greet you differently from the way they greeted your brothers? For example, did they shake hands with your brother, and then bounce, kiss, and squeeze you and otherwise physically condition you to be passive while you were with men? (There is nothing at all against lots of physical warmth, but especially at family gatherings it can be excessive.) Was your brother openly favored? Or you? Were you given housework while your brother helped your father fix things?

Was your mother ashamed to tell you about menstruation? What did your mother say about sex to you—did she treat it as something to fear? As something dirty? Painful? Joyful? Something *she* wanted? Something men need? Was she ashamed if you didn't date? If you weren't popular? If you were overweight? If you were a tomboy, what was your parents' reaction? For example, did they openly express hope that you'd "grow out of it" and be "boy-crazy," given time? Were your parents afraid that you would be a lesbian if you refused to abandon "masculine" pursuits and adopt ladylike, "feminine" behavior and interests?

Did your mother look forward to your wedding for years in advance, urging you, for example, to pick out silver and china patterns? How did your parents refer to single women? Childless women? Were you told that high school was enough for a girl? Or, were you allowed to go to college to get a "safety backup," just in case? Did the family sacrifice to push your brother, not you, ahead? How were your ambitions treated?

Were your parents happily married? Separated? Divorced? Do you know why? Did your mother have to make it alone? Did your mother sacrifice *all* her time for children? Did she work outside the home? Was she passive? Was she helpless about mechanical or financial things? Did she make fun of herself? Did she pick on your father? Did she envy your father? Was she often depressed? On tranquilizers or therapists? Did she drink alone? Did she have affairs? Did you ever feel you wanted to be like her or not like her?

The point of asking questions like these is not to find out whether you secretly hate or love or love/hate your mother and father, or whether they gave your psyche some neurotic complex. It's not to place blame either—pointing a finger will not by itself help you handle your present problems with strength. The point of such questions is to see if they shed any light on how you are responding to the restraints you face as a woman in the present—the kinds of demands made of you that might be creating massive waves of self-loathing, depression, even madness. Figuring out your problems with a therapist may involve two kinds of questions: (1) Those having to do with the pressures and contradictions that have set the framework of your life as a woman now, and (2) those having to do with the attitudes and expectations about women and men you have internalized as you were growing up. Once understanding these two sources of your difficulties, you and your therapist may be able to work out a way for you to fight back with self-confidence and independence.

NORMS OF "FEMININITY"

Cultural stereotypes of women are numerous, but perhaps the most fundamental ones that have seriously affected many therapists emerge from the belief that the psychology of men and women is inherently different. Different bodies make different minds. Anatomy is destiny. Your body's sexual and reproductive organs determine for you a whole set of psychological qualities and roles that you should attempt to fulfill. Women should strive to be "feminine," and "femininity" means being soft, emotional, intuitive, sensitive, childlike, passive, submissive, giving, loving, and sympathetic—all qualities supposedly best suited to the home. Men should be "masculine," and "masculinity" in our culture means being powerful, strong, directed, intellectual, capable of abstract reasoning, aggressive, assertive, mechanical, sexually potent, muscular, athletic, and blunt—all qualities thought necessary for achievement in the world *beyond* the home.

If you show "feminine" qualities, your therapist is likely to be supportive and encouraging. If you show "masculine" qualities, your therapist may question you sharply and try to undermine your typical ways of thinking and behaving. Even if he or she accepts your "masculine" characteristics, a sharp division between you and other "feminine" women is likely to be made. Your therapist might stress, for example, that if you continue in your independent ways, you will be very threatening to men, and it will be unlikely you will ever have successful love relationships.

Phyllis Chesler, in *Women and Madness*, quoted a woman she interviewed:

[My boyfriend] suggested I see his psychiatrist, a man. So I did. He kept saying that I should wear my hair long instead of pulled back because it was more feminine. But it got tangled in fifteen minutes and I couldn't stand it. And he told me to put no pressure on my boy friend . . . he told me to just be "giving" for a change. At the time I was very afraid that the things he was saying were true—even though

I would fight with him. There must be something wrong with a woman being assertive, intelligent and capable. I was, and no one was loving me very much, and I was very unhappy.[1]

Like anyone else, your therapist may or may not be aware of the operation of these stereotypes in his or her response to you and your problems. But unless he/she has consciously struggled against these attitudes that so permeate our culture, it is very likely they will play some part in your therapy—maybe a very destructive part.

Many therapists like to believe they are completely objective and value-free, that they only want to help you grow in whatever direction you choose. In such a case, it may be particularly difficult to avoid being overwhelmed by the therapist's belief in his/her own scientific objectivity. Other therapists are now recognizing that they are human beings first and foremost and that they cannot, therefore, escape their own values and categories about women and men. With a therapist like this, it may be easier for you to escape the rigid division between "femininity" and "masculinity" that is so oppressive and limiting for both women and men.

If you are in therapy now, ask yourself what assumptions your therapist has about women and men, "femininity" and "masculinity." Ask yourself particularly if he or she puts you into either of the two basic categories we describe in the following two sections.

The "Feminine Woman"

Here is Hélène Deutsch's description of typical "feminine" women:

> To the [feminine] woman falls the larger share of the work of adjustment: she leaves the initiative to the man and out of her own need renounces originality, experiencing her own self through identification.... These women are not only ideal life companions for men; they possess the feminine quality of intuition to a great degree, they are ideal collaborators who often inspire their men, and are them-

selves happiest in this role. They seem to be easily influenceable, and adapt themselves to their companions and understand them. They are the loveliest and most unaggressive of helpmates and they want to remain in that role; they do not insist on their own rights—quite the contrary. They are easy to handle in every way—if one only loves them. Sexually, they are easily excited and rarely frigid; but precisely in that sexual field they impose narcissistic conditions which must be fulfilled absolutely. They demand love and ardent desire, finding in these a satisfying compensation for the renunication of their own active tendencies.

If gifted in any direction, they preserve the capacity for being original and productive, but without entering into competitive struggles. They are always willing to renounce their own achievements without feeling that they are sacrificing anything and they rejoice in the achievements of their companions, which they have often inspired. They have an extraordinary need of support when engaged in any *activity directed outward*, but are absolutely independent in such thinking and feeling as relate to their inner life, that is to say, in their *activity directed inward*. Their capacity for identification is not an expression of inner poverty, but of inner wealth.[2]

This is Hélène Deutsch's description of the ideal "feminine woman"; this stereotype of the woman who may be intelligent and creative, but also easily "influenceable" and undemanding of her rights is an extremely familiar one. Its ideal is completely inapplicable to the growing numbers of women who are heads of household—whether from poverty, choice, divorce, or death. But it is fed to us from childhood on through adulthood by the media, by the educational system, and by the women we have as models around us. And as Seymour Halleck has written: "The founders of psychoanalysis saw women as basically masochistic and passive—as needing a certain degree of masculine domination in order to feel comfortable and whole."[3] It should be no surprise that such psychological theories are subtly incorporated into many therapists' models of the well-adjusted female.

Because the "feminine" woman has both desirable and undesirable qualities, she is difficult to dissect. The negative side of the "feminine woman" is characterized not by what she is, but by what she *isn't. She isn't original*—she can't come up with new solutions to her problems. *She is not strong-willed*—even if she does come up with a new idea, she doesn't have enough faith in her own ability and must constantly be reassured. *She is not rational or realistic*—in intellectual matters, she can't divorce herself from her emotions. *She is not decisive*—she needs others to make her decisions for her. *She is not dependable*—she falls apart in a crisis. *She is not a leader*—how can she be, when she's lacking all these qualities? *She is not sexually aggressive*—she must wait for a man to initiate a relationship.

The "feminine woman" is not supposed to be *physically skilled*—her body has been developed for beauty, not for utility. *She isn't mechanical or scientific*—she can't do anything requiring these qualities. She is usually trapped into traditional "care-giving" feminine occupations (extensions of women's traditional roles) without being able to exercise choice. All together, these qualities make her depend on others for shelter, food, and clothing as well as for a reason for living.

The qualities which we in this book call "desirable" in the "feminine woman" are not viewed as desirable by society in general and men in particular because these qualities are associated with weakness. We think of them as strengths. The "feminine woman" is *cooperative*—her interactions mainly involve working *with* people, not competing against them. *She realizes when other people's needs must come first*—her life is not totally self-centered. *She is supportive*—she doesn't see other people's achievements as a threat. *She is sympathetic*—she can identify with the problems of others. *She is in touch with her emotions*—she is not openly afraid of expressing "joy" or "sadness" and she freely expresses warmth and affection. *She is willing to admit she's wrong*—her ego is not so frail that she must be right all the time.

If these qualities were not her whole self, but one important part of her personality, they would not be called weak by the rest of society. Just because she is supportive, cooperative, and sympathetic doesn't mean that she cannot also be decisive, mechanical, sexually assertive, and a leader. The therapist's notion of the woman's role in society and the woman's notion of her own role do not have to involve a choice between two polar opposites. Neither the therapist nor the woman has to reject all of the qualities associated with "femininity." Instead, they can choose the best qualities and make them an integral part of an otherwise independent life.

The "Masculine Woman"

Women who are active, assertive, openly intelligent, ambitious, full of opinions about things, athletic, scientific, and mechanical are not likely to be awarded any prizes for being "feminine" in our society. Women who reject marriage or children are simply "unfeminine." And the femininity of women who insist on working, on financial independence, on having friends of their own in addition to husband, lover, or children is always a matter for debate. A woman with these qualities, interests, and desires would be considered "healthy" or "normal" if she were a man. But because she is a woman, these qualities suddenly make her "sick" or "maladjusted."

Matina Horner wrote:

> As a whole, society has been unable to reconcile personal ambition with femininity. The more successful or independent a woman becomes, the more afraid society is that she has lost her femininity and therefore must be a failure as a wife and mother. She is viewed as a hostile and destructive force within the society. On the other hand, the more successful a man is in his work (as reflected in his high status, salary and administrative powers—all of which are in keeping with his masculinity), the more attractive he becomes as a spouse and father. Whereas men are unsexed by failure . . . women seem to be unsexed by success.[4]

In terms of the prevailing stereotypes of our culture, such a woman is not a "real woman"; she is a "masculine woman." Her dissatisfaction with the traditionally feminine role is a sign of a "masculinity complex."

For example, in Doris Lessing's novel *The Four-Gated City*, a psychiatrist tells Martha, the main character:

> I think you are proud of your knowing—you are proud of that more than anything. It's your intelligence you are proud of. You are still fighting your mother with that—the masculine intelligence.[5]

An independent woman is considered by many to be a great threat to the sensitive male ego. One psychologist wrote in a *New York Times Magazine* article that women connected to the woman's movement posed a serious and unfair threat to male sexuality. Male potency is so delicately vulnerable, he argued, that assertive women would make sex (and ultimately the human race) impossible (translation: since men are weak, women must let them have all the power!).

This threatening quality of the "masculine woman" is said to make her "castrating." Her strength emasculates men, crucifies them. She is the "Bitch," the "Witch." And obviously, she can never have a satisfying sexual relationship with a man—or so the stereotype would have it. The man connected with such a woman is often the object of covert derision—by virtue of his relationship with her he must be "emasculated," "hen-pecked."

Her independence is threatening not only in bed but also in work and friendship. Many jobs are closed to her, and she is genuinely disliked and feared by many for qualities that would be considered positive in a man. This was the experience of one woman we interviewed:

> *I had been seeing a therapist privately for some time. One day he had me join a group session with some other people and his co-therapist. My therapist said to his partner that I was very threatening to him because I was so bright. This admission seems honest enough, but in private with me, he was always cutting down my dedication to graduate study and teaching. He told me that my working so hard was just part of my craziness.*

Even where the "masculine woman" is accepted as she is, the assumption of many around her is that she is still "unfeminine" and "cold"—shut off from the capacity to give and receive love.

If your therapist has internalized society's antagonism against this type of independent woman, he or she may decide you are in danger of becoming a "masculine woman" when you show signs of defiance against traditional "femininity." Cynthia Cekala quoted a woman who had been in a mental hospital:

> The one girl of my building I was friends with usually went to bed at six o'clock since she was on very heavy medication. Sometimes I would go to her room or she to mine and we would talk. My doctor accused me of having a lesbian relationship with her. Throughout my stay there I wore what I had worn at school—boots and jeans and sweaters. The shrink told me that if I didn't give up being a hippie and wear skirts I could not be considered to be cured. In my record, I was "masculine." It was at this session that he asked me if I was a lesbian. My friend was also warned that if she hung around me it was sure to be a bad influence.[6]

In an attempt to help you avoid this "deviance" from the accepted norm, your therapist may support your passive tendencies and attack your active qualities and "masculine" interests, as Halleck observed:

> A woman who enters psychotherapy will usually be exposed to a system of values that emphasizes the virtues of passivity; if she rejects these values her therapist may interpret her attitude as immature.[7]

If your therapist is a man, he may in fact be personally threatened by any assertiveness on your part against him, his ideas, or his authority.

DOUBLE STANDARDS FOR "MENTAL HEALTH": A VOCABULARY GUIDE FOR SEXIST SHRINKS *

If a "Patient" Is	She Is	He Is
PASSIVE	SWEET	CASTRATED
TOUGH	AGGRESSIVE	GO-GETTER, AMBITIOUS
SUPPORTIVE	UNDERSTANDING	YES-MAN
INTELLIGENT	TOO SMART FOR HER OWN GOOD	INTELLIGENT
INDEPENDENT	FRUSTRATED	INDEPENDENT
A LEADER	CASTRATING	DECISIVE
INNOVATIVE	PUSHY	ORIGINAL
INSISTENT	HYSTERICAL	PERSISTENT
CUTE, TIMID	A SWEETHEART	HOMOSEXUAL
PLAIN-LOOKING	LETTING HERSELF GO	NO COMMENT
SUCCESSFUL	BALL-BREAKER	SUCCESSFUL
POLITICALLY INVOLVED	OVER-EMOTIONAL	COMMITTED
SUPPORTIVE, HELPFUL, INGRATIATING, PASSIVE, GENTLE	A REAL WOMAN	A NOTHING

*With help from "How to Name Baby—A Vocabulary Guide for Working Women," by Media Women, printed in **Sisterhood is Powerful**, Robin Morgan, ed. (New York: Random House, 1970), pp. 526–27.

Androgynous Womanhood

Some nontraditional therapists today, especially feminist therapists, have abandoned the belief that men and women must be psychological opposites. The differences that do exist between men and women, they argue, are largely the result of the socialization of children into "masculine" and "feminine" adults. Women and men have the potential to become whole human beings, each one synthesizing within herself or himself the best qualities traditionally associated with masculinity" and "femininity." Psychologist Sandra Bem has conducted studies showing that the "healthiest" or strongest people are "androgynous" (from the Greek roots, *andro*—man, *gyne*—woman).[8] They have the capacity to be both nurturing and independent, both supportive and achieving, both active and receptive. For women, this idea of androgyny holds out a potential alternative to the culture's separation of women into "feminine" women and "masculine" women. There is often a conflict of seemingly mutually exclusive desires at the root of women's depression: Should I be a wife and mother? Should I get training for a career? Should I stay at home with my kids? Should I work outside the home? Do the man's needs always come before my own? I'm the "head of household;" but can I be a "real woman" too? The idea of androgyny sets forth a possible resolution of these dilemmas by suggesting that sex roles should be eliminated and that psychological identity should allow a full range of human potential. Relationships between women and men, parents and children, employers and employees should be changed so that no woman (or man) is forced into an exclusively "masculine" or "feminine" mold, so that women have the chance to be fully human.

You may not have heard the term "androgyny" before, but the concept is familiar to many psychologists because of wide circulation of Sandra Bem's (and other feminist psychologists') work. As a way of evaluating your therapist, you could ask him/her whether he/she is open to the idea of changing current concepts of sex roles and male and female identity. Your therapist's response might be a good touchstone.

THE LESBIAN IN THERAPY*

Lesbians come in all sizes, shapes, attitudes, and social classes. But, if you tell your therapist you are a lesbian and you do not fit the old-line stereotypes, be ready for, "But you don't look like one!"

The old-line stereotypes dictate that a lesbian be in one of two types. The "butch" or "bull-dyke" is a woman who has

---

*This section has been written for the book by Victoria Cazel. She attended a few meetings with our group for a short period, read our drafts, participated in some of our discussions, and wrote "The Lesbian in Therapy" for the book. With her permission, we have interspersed as extracts the comments of people we interviewed and other pertinent quoted material. Thus the material set off from the text in this section is our addition, with Victoria Cazel's knowledge and permission.

become a caricature of a man. She wears a black leather jacket, old blue jeans, a sweatshirt, and boots. Her hair is cut short, and her language is foul. She is too heavy, too tall, too athletic, too ugly, and too independent to catch a man. She may, at one time, have been spurned by a man, and she is bitter. She wants to avenge herself, and she treats women badly. Sometimes she is even said to seduce virgins. When she has made love to one of these poor virgins, the woman she has seduced can never be satisfied by a man. Her sex life consists of brutal, abrupt, short-term *attacks* on other women. She straps on a dildo (penis substitute) and screws the other woman into submission. Or, she produces her whip collection and beats her partner mercilessly. She finds her sex partners in back-alley bars or in public restrooms. All her relationships last about one night. The butch can never be satisfied sexually. She gains her pleasure from violence, but never has an orgasm; this further frustrates her and moves her to more violence.

A psychiatrist, Alexander Lowen, has a chapter in his book *Love and Orgasm* called "The Lesbian Personality." In it, he discusses the cases of a number of lesbians who came to him for therapy. His discussion shows that he accepts the common division of lesbians into two personality types, one aggressive and the other passive. He writes: "In appearance, the typical masculine female is quite imposing. She has a large body, broad shoulders, a short neck, and a rather big head with strong features. She tends to be brusque and hard. She knows her business, and she knows what she wants. In manner and attitude, she is the successful executive. . . . The masculine female usually attracts a soft, dependent, feminine type of homosexual in lesbian relationships." His descriptions of individual lesbians are not as simplistic as this introductory statement—for example, he notes that Debora, one of the "butch" lesbians, had a phsycial appearance that "impressed" him "as resembling a gorilla"; but she also "revealed an inner sensitivity that belied her outward appearance." Nonetheless, Lowen continues to see lesbians in two basic categories that he calls "masculine" and "feminine."[9]

The second type is the butch's partner, the "femme." The femme is a caricature of a woman. She wears super-feminine clothes, too much makeup, and constantly acts in a seductive manner. She is a divorcee or a woman who has had a bad experience with a man, she is a virgin afraid of pregnancy, or she is a prostitute who gives her body to men for business and to women for pleasure. The femme is also interested more in short-term relationships than long-term relationships. The femme is greatly aroused by violence and is proud when she hooks a butch with a bad reputation. The femme, since she is very feminine, catches the eyes of both men and women. She derives much pleasure from leading men on.

According to the stereotypes, both types of women, butch and femme, come from the lower and working classes. There are no middle- or upper-class lesbians. There are also no lesbians in the suburbs or rural areas; they all gather in the worst parts of the big cities. The stereotypical relationship is always violent and more than likely, mocks the roles of heterosexuality.

> From an interview with a lesbian: *"When I told my therapist I was gay, he laughed. I come from a good family, live in the suburbs, and was a college student. It was just a phase . . . he said."*

Fortunately, these stereotypes are fading. Lesbians of the forties and fifties often did take on the stereotypical roles, but even then, long-term relationships were very common. One-night stands in bars or bathrooms have never been a common lesbian practice.

Lesbian use of dildos is just another fantasy of a sexist society in which men cannot comprehend how a woman can be satisfied without a penis.

> From an interview: *"After my therapist found out I was a lesbian, he asked me endlessly what I did in bed. He asked me whether my lover and I used a dildo, and what did it look like. I told him I had never seen a dildo. He looked baffled . . . and upset."*

In actuality, the dildo is more likely to be used by a hetero-sexual woman in masturbation. Sadism and masochism are not common lesbian practices, and never have been. Violence is usually associated with frustration to an extreme. Lesbian relationships are no more fraught with frustration than any other intimate relationship in this society. Lesbian relation-ships are characterized, just as all other intimate relation-ships, with caring, loving, and tenderness.

Don't let a therapist dismiss you by placing you in one of the convenient stereotypes and declaring you "sick."

> From personal correspondence with a lesbian: "*While I was moping around at school I got to talking with this older woman whom I had always considered to be an unreformed 60's radical, always ready with the right rhetoric and she told me that she had been in therapy for seven years. She said that her male therapist had told her that her lesbianism was the only proper political response to the sexism of the last four decades. . . . I consider him a star on the horizon, a lone star.*"

Lowen's concluding paragraph in his chapter "The Lesbian Personality" from *Love and Orgasm* clearly expresses the assumption that heterosexuality, as opposed to homosexu-ality, is a norm for mental health: "We must accept the homo-sexual, if we are to help him. This does not mean that we should approve of his behavior. It does mean that we should try to understand his desperate need to find someone to love. His desire for physical closeness to another in no way differs from that of the normal person. However, his ability to ex-press those feelings is severely limited. For love can be fully expressed only in a heterosexual relationship, which for the homosexual is so charged with guilt that it is a closed door." Lowen continues by saying that the homosexual's need for love does find some outlet "with the homosexual despising the person he needs and hating himself for the need." He con-cludes with, "What a tragic way to live! What a limitation of the potential of the human personality!"[10]

Phyllis Chesler, in her book *Women and Madness*, quoted a woman's description of her therapist's reaction when she told him she was a lesbian:

> "He freaked out. He started yelling at me. 'You're doing this because you think I'm your father and you want to hurt your father. You're a spoiled child!' ... and he just freaked me out! Y'know. Because, since I'd been in therapy, I was truly happy. I did what I wanted to do, 'n she was really lovely, and I was very happy. ... He sort of made me understand that it was a very unfortunate thing that I was doing and that it would result in heartache. Which I understand, I mean, I do. It's certainly much better to live within the system. ... Then he said, 'How could you stand it—don't women smell awful?' ... and I said, 'I don't know, it just doesn't bother me.' 'Did you ever see the statue of David?' he said. 'A man's body is so much more beautiful than a woman's body!' ... 'You're crazy,' I said. 'I'm not saying my values are *the* values, but you better dig it, Doctor, and check out your own set of eyes, you've got some thinking to do.' "[11]

Education of your therapist is an important factor; you can suggest that he/she read any of the several excellent books that are being written by, for, and about lesbians. Finally, if you are unsure about your sexuality, beware of the therapist who will try to "push" you either into heterosexuality or homosexuality. Ultimately, you must answer to no one but yourself, so go along with your feelings and emotions.

Victoria Cazel's conclusion about the need of women in therapy to determine an identity, lifestyle, and sexual orientation that are centered in their own feelings rather than in any externally imposed norm can usefully apply to all women in therapy—no matter what issues they are discussing. Whatever role conflicts you are facing, however uncertain you are about the meaning of "womanhood," be critical of a therapist who imposes ready-made diagnoses, identities, and solutions for your difficulties. A good therapist *can* be a rich resource of experience, challenging (even tough or painful) questions, perceptive interpretations, and ideas for your range of options.

But a therapist who hands you a solution to your problems without engaging you in the process of thinking for yourself is not likely to help you develop independence or confidence in your own potential for growth. The importance of the therapist's respect for your perspective and needs is especially crucial in the subject of the next chapter—female sexuality.

FOOTNOTES

[1]Phyllis Chesler, *Women and Madness* (New York: Doubleday, 1972), pp. 256-57. Excerpts from *Women and Madness* by Phyllis Chesler. Copyright © 1972 by Phyllis Chesler. Reprinted by permission of Doubleday & Company, Inc. and Penguin Books Ltd.

[2]Hélène Deutsch, *The Psychology of Women*, Vol. I (New York: Grune & Stratton, 1944), pp. 191-92. Used by permission of Hélène Deutsch and Grune & Stratton.

[3]Seymour Halleck, *Politics of Therapy* (New York: Science House, 1971), p. 109.

[4]Matina S. Horner, "Femininity and Successful Achievement: A Basic Incongruity," in *Roles Women Play: Readings Toward Women's Liberation*, Michelle Hoffnung Garskof, ed. (Belmont, Cal.: Brooks/Cole, 1971), p. 106.

[5]From Doris Lessing's *The Four-Gated City* (New York: Knopf, 1969), p. 241.

[6]Cynthia Cekala, "If This Be Insanity . . .", *Rough Times*, 3, no. 1 (September 1972), 2. *Rough Times* was first called *The Radical Therapist* and is now called *State and Mind*.

[7]Halleck, *Politics of Therapy*, p. 109.

[8]See, for example, Sandra L. Bem, "Probing the Promise of Androgyny," in *Beyond Sex-Role Stereotypes: Readings Toward a Psychology of Androgyny*, Alexandra G. Kaplan and Joan P. Bean, eds. (Boston: Little, Brown and Co., 1976), pp. 47-62. See also Alexandra Kaplan's excellent "Androgyny as a Model of Mental Health for Women: From Theory to Therapy," in the same volume, pp. 352-62.

[9]Alexander Lowen, *Love and Orgasm* (New York: Macmillan, 1975), p. 86.

[10]Ibid., p. 107. The issue of whether or not homosexuality is a mental illness has been seriously debated in the medical profession in recent years. In 1973, the American Psychiatric Association voted by a narrow margin that homosexuality is *not* a mental illness. While this vote is of great importance in the future training of therapists, such a vote is not likely to change overnight the attitudes of therapists who have seen homosexuality as a form of illness or deviance. This is especially true since the vote does not reflect the widespread homophobia (fear of homosexuality) current in the United States today. With the impact of the gay rights movement, some therapists may no longer say blatantly that homosexuality is deviant. But when conscious or unconscious prejudice goes underground, it has the potential to shape the course of therapy even more subtly and insidiously.

[11]Chesler, *Women and Madness*, p. 195.

The Therapist and Female Sexuality

Sexuality is one of the most crucial issues concerning women in therapy. Although all the women in our group could easily agree on that, we found ourselves continually putting off writing this chapter. It took a long time for us to admit that the reason for our procrastination was that it meant exposing a part of our lives to each other—a part that we were unsure of and were in some ways ashamed of. Even though the subjects of the other sections touched us very personally, nothing touched us as deeply as the topic of our own sexuality. We realized that we have internalized all the myths society has built up around women and sexuality. And, since our personal experiences do not fit with those myths, each of us thought that there must be something wrong with us; and that was painful and difficult to admit. Our first discussions were filled with nervous laughter and uncomfortable silences. Eventually we began to open up. We discovered that although no two of us had identical experiences, we all had one thing in common—we were all contradictions to society's myths of "normal" female sexuality. Most of us rarely had orgasms during intercourse (when the penis is in the vagina); we all experienced orgasms differently; and we all had different feelings about and experience with masturbation.

It felt good to talk about our fears and realize that they weren't the result of our individual inadequacies, but instead were created by our socialization and perpetuated by our isolation from one another.

We don't think our experience is unique. We think most women are struggling with the same problems and are unable to open up. Many are desperately unhappy, partly because their sexual lives offer them not pleasure, but frustration and guilt. They can't bring themselves to talk to friends or lovers about their feelings, so they become lonely and isolated with no way out of their depression. They believe that they are so maladjusted that if they open up, others might attack and totally reject them.

A woman who feels this way is especially vulnerable to a therapist who believes society's myths. Such a therapist will reinforce all her fears by telling her that the sexual ideal she can't adjust to is the only one worth striving for. Because she isn't talking to anyone else about her feelings, the power of the therapist is multiplied.

We think one first step toward learning how to attain sexual fulfillment is to get together with other women and talk, listen, and share. It may not be the *only* first step for women. But by talking to one another, maybe we will discover there is no "normal" female sexuality—whatever we feel comfortable with, whatever gives us emotional and physical pleasure, and whichever sex we are attracted to is okay. It is okay as long as we have the freedom to discover it for ourselves and are not forced into the "happiness" of a traditional, passive, male-centered sexual relationship. We can do better than that.

BODY THOUGHTS

You are ugly. You are fat. Your breasts are too small (or large). Your thighs are too fat, your calves are too thin. Your eyes are too small. Your hair is mousy-colored. Your nose has a bump. You are too skinny. You have hair on your face. Your hair is too curly. Your hair is too thin. You have midriff bulge. You have vaginal odor. You wear glasses. Your face is covered with pimples. You compare yourself to almost every woman you see, even ones you just pass on the street. If you're comparing hips, and yours are larger than hers, for a second you hate your body; if yours are smaller than hers, you feel relief. After all, if a man came by and had to choose between the two of you, he would prefer you, because you have smaller hips. The process goes on, but no matter who you compare yourself with, you never really feel good about your body.

> I am the plain Jane of the family and just long for beauty. When I go to the pictures and see the beautiful girls it makes me cry to think I'm so unattractive. Can you give me any beauty hints?[1]

The amazing thing is that every woman we know feels (or has felt) the same way, including those who fit the accepted or currently fashionable definition of "beautiful." Women have been taught to hate their bodies. We spend hours trying to change ourselves, and even if we have gotten away from wearing makeup, and changing our hair color, we spend hours hating what we are and wishing we looked different. Psychologists have long noted women's obsession with the seeming inadequacies of their bodies. Freud's theory of female psychosexual development, in fact, rests on his attempt to explain women's insecurity about their body. He theorized that both women's "vanity" (or "narcissim") and modesty (or "shame") arose as compensation for "genital deficiency." In comparison to the male physiology, women were indeed inferior in Freud's view. Recognition of that anatomical inadequacy is thus a crucial moment in a girl's psychological development. He wrote for example:

> the discovery that she is castrated is a turning point in a girl's growth.
> ... Her self-love is mortified by the comparison with the boy's far superior equipment.[2]

Where *does* women's insecurity about their bodies come from: Is Freud correct in believing that men's bodies are inherently superior? We don't think so. Instead, we suggest that women often experience their bodies as they appear in men's eyes. When men think of women, many think of bodies—their beauty and potential value for sex (or lack of it). A young girl might think of herself as a whole person, but as she becomes a woman she learns that the man's point of view is the only one that counts. So she learns to think of herself and other women as "bodies." She accepts the idea that a woman is valued for what she looks like, while a man is valued for what he *does*. Someone summed up the situation in an airlines magazine: "A woman's face is her fortune. A man's face is his life."

Once a woman accepts this idea, she is open to many forms of self-disgust. She is bombarded with standards of beauty via television, magazines, and other media. It doesn't matter what the current standard of beauty is—the only qualification is that it be unattainable. This unattainable standard is created at the whim of business*men* who run the industries that prey on women—the fashion industry, the cosmetics industry, the diet industry (diet foods, health clubs, etc.). These standards are consciously designed to be unattainable. If they weren't, how could the industries make their millions? A woman's body becomes just another case of planned obsolescence. Once a woman accepts the fact that this Madison Avenue man's point of view is the only one, she can experience only frustration and self-hate about her body.

The destructiveness of these unattainable standards reaches a whole new dimension for Black, Asian, Indian, and many Jewish and Latin women—in short, for any woman of a cultural group that has distinctive physiological characteristics. The ideal of the beautiful woman *none* of us ever looks like places a double burden on women of different races, for that plastic, nonexistent model spread all over the world by Hollywood and fashion magazines is *white*—and often blond and blue-eyed. Women born with dark or black skin, thick lips, kinky hair, Semitic noses, Asian eyelids (and so on and on) all too often have internalized a standard of beauty that comes from the majority culture. The result: hair straighteners, nose jobs, eye operations, and skin-bleaching creams—all in the attempt to remake the body. Implicit in such an attempt is a negative body image originating in the majority culture. Implicit also is the belief that the very *genetic* make-up of the woman's racial group can never measure up to that unattainable ideal of "beauty."

I am white, and I was teaching a nearly all-Black college literature class. We were discussing Malcolm X's story of his first conk [hair straightening]. Every woman and every man in that class said that they could not respect a man today who straightened his hair—he had no pride in his race, they said. I was stunned at first, because as I looked around the room, over half of the women had straightened hair—typical of the whole college and the subway crowd, as I began to notice. My students explained that women need to have a variety of hairstyles to be fashionable, that Afros take a lot of work, that your hair falls out, etc. There were a dozen reasons why women should straighten their hair if they wanted to, although I couldn't see why all these reasons, except the "fashion" one, wouldn't apply to men as well. My students were crystal-clear—a man shows no race pride if he straightens his hair, but a woman doesn't lower herself by doing so. I can't help wondering if some of the white standards are still binding the Black women while the men have become more liberated as far as appearance goes. How many Asian men slit their eyelids? How many Jewish men have nose jobs? Acceptable beauty is not a man's ticket to a happy future. How much have things really changed for minority women?

The recent rejection of white standards by nonwhite peoples has helped reverse this kind of racist socialization process. But while one racial burden is lifted, how about that primary burden—of being a woman whose worth is measured in terms of her body? What happens to the Black woman who doesn't meet the new Black standard for beauty? Or the Asian woman? Or the Indian? If a woman still feels underneath it all that her future depends on what she looks like, how much does it matter that one unattainable standard for beauty has been replaced by another? She may still end up feeling frustrated and worthless.

This frustration about surface appearance often parallels an even deeper disgust with the natural smells and processes of our bodies. Menstruation is a dark secret—in many places packages of tampons and sanitary pads are still placed in plain brown paper bags like the covers of a pornographic book. Even where menstruation is more openly referred to, taboos against intercourse during a woman's period are still widespread. Germaine Greer, in *The Female Eunuch*,[3] asks which one of us can taste a drop of menstrual blood the way we can blood from a pin prick on the finger. Hair on legs, underarms, and faces—all signs of potent sexuality on a man—are carefully and sometimes painfully eliminated as if we fear any outward show of our own sexuality. Advertising for "feminine hygiene" spray has resulted in an instantaneously successful industry, for it builds on our fears that our sexual organs are fundamentally revolting unless they are sterilized, cleaned up, powdered over, prepared, and made enticing like the rest of our body by strawberry, lime, or raspberry perfume.

Internalization of loathing or shame for women's genitals has greatly inhibited the full expression of female sexuality—for both heterosexual and lesbian women. A woman told us:

> *My feelings about oral sex are very ambivalent. I love the feeling of my husband's tongue and breath—it's totally different, delicate, yet intense, sometimes excruciating. But if I haven't taken a shower right before we make love, I get very tense and so embarrassed that I can't say a word; excitement often vanishes. I know I feel embarrassed by how I smell, and I know that this disgust comes originally from the culture. I have always been deeply insulted by these 'inti-*

mate' sprays and would never use one. But the problem seems to be getting worse.

Freud's belief that the snake-covered head of Medusa (which turns anyone who dares to look upon it to stone) is the mythic symbol for our genitals does capture something of the hidden fears about our bodies we often live with. But while he thought this disgust to be rationally and objectively justified, we see it as the painful result of how we are directly and indirectly taught to think of ourselves.

You may talk to your therapist about your dissatisfaction with your body. There are several responses he or she could have to the feelings you express. Your therapist could tell you that your feelings about the way you look are a symptom of your obsessive-compulsive neurosis—in other words, you love to worry, and there is no real problem. One woman we interviewed said:

> *I saw a woman therapist once, and told her that I was upset because I thought men looked at me all the time—looked at my breasts and the way I walked, in a very sex-object fashion. She asked me, "Why don't you just enjoy it?"*

We don't think this is a fair response. Your feelings have been brought about by a real situation—you need only listen to the women around you to see that your feelings are mirrored in all of them.

Another negative way your therapist could respond to your feelings would be to say, "If you think you are ugly, *do* something about it. Change your hairstyle, buy new clothes, fix yourself up."

> "Why don't you fix yourself up?" [the therapist] always said. "You look like a hobo—I'd almost think you were afraid of men!" Not a word about how right we are to be afraid. Not a word about athletics, lesbianism, politics or my eternal soul, just "Dress up for Daddy" as proof of mental health.[4]

I had a doctor who kept interviewing me. He'd go over the same story over and over again. I remember I was looking terrible, my hair wasn't combed, I had no makeup. He said, "Why don't you fix yourself up? A nice girl like you!" And I said, "I never want another man to look at me again."[5]

Your therapist is responding according to the way he or she has been socialized. Therapists' feelings are likely to be a reflection of all the attitudes about women that made you feel repulsive in the first place. They are apt to see you as a "body" first of all like the rest of the world. Therefore, their suggestions are not going to help you.

You might get another kind of response from a therapist with heavy psychoanalytic training. He or she might see your worries about your body as a sign of the narcissism that is supposedly a basic characteristic of all women. Freud said that this narcissism was simply justified overcompensation for a genuine anatomical inferiority to men. (That is, you don't have a penis, you feel bad about it, and so you get either negatively or positively fascinated with your own body to compensate for your lack of the "superior equipment"—that's really what Freud called the penis—of men.) In this context, your therapist may see your worry as an exaggeration to the point of neurosis of a basically healthy, "feminine" narcissism. This kind of therapist puts your concern and self-consciousness into a psychological, purely personal framework instead of viewing your feelings as the product of cultural attitudes and the economics of the cosmetic and fashion industries.

This response—that narcissism is necessary for *female* mental health as opposed to the energetic aggressiveness ideal for the "healthy" male—permeates the discussion of Black women and men in *Black Rage,* a book by two Black psychiatrists. In their chapter on "Acquiring Manhood," Grier and Cobbs say that white society (and Black mothers) have taken away the Black male's ability to reach for power and money, to exercise the "certain prerogatives and privileges" of men, to be "assertive" and "aggressive." Not a word about narcissism. This lid on the development of Black manhood must be lifted if Black men are to avoid a general, socially created neurosis.[6] How can Black women be saved? In their chapter entitled "Achieving Womanhood," Grier and Cobbs' answer is much more rigidly Freudian than was Freud's own counsel to his women analysands. Black women, the authors say, must be taught that they are beautiful (if they are among those whose "feminine narcissism [can] rest ultimately on real physical attractiveness"[7]). Black women are victims of white standards of beauty. The Black woman "has derived none of the intensely personal satisfaction she might have received as an honored and desirable sex object."[8]

Her road to liberation is pride in her "African features," a sense that she is "an especially worthwhile person," i.e., *she has achieved a "healthy narcissism."*[9] Not a word about a woman's need for growth and pride in *any* other dimension but the world of love and sex! They are of course correct that Black women have been severely victimized by white standards of beauty. They argue correctly that Black women and men should reject the white norms for hair, skin color, features, and body structure. But they continue to teach that a woman's confidence and self-worth rest fundamentally on her narcissism—on her ability to feel like a "desirable sex object." How she should feel about herself if she is not "beautiful" by Afro-American standards is never discussed. How she is to explore aspects of her identity outside of her sexuality is never addressed. Like so many other therapists, Cobbs and Grier have totally different ideas for mental health in men and women. Black men will assert their manhood through the power and achievements so long denied them by white society. Black women will discover their womanhood through affirmation of their sexuality. The category "human being" doesn't seem to exist.

Again quoting from Grier and Cobbs:

> Anatomy determines that every girl will struggle with feelings of having been injured and mutilated when she compares her sexual organs with the male's, but under normal circumstances the compensatory blossoming of narcissism allows her to develop a feeling of

satisfaction with herself. The black woman's feelings of mutilation, both psychical and physical, are strengthened by her experiences and she is guarded from self-depreciation only by an enfeebled narcissism. As a result, her personal ambitions as an adolescent and her capacity to live out her aspirations suffer. . . . With youthful narcissism crushed and sexual life perverted, [Black women] drew back from these modes as primary means of life expression. Letting youth go, beauty go, and sex go, they narrowed their vision to the most essential feminine functioning—mothering, nurturing, and protecting their children.[10]

If your therapist doesn't try to change you from a Cinderella in rags to a beautiful princess, you may be lucky enough to meet with a third kind of response. Your therapist could make a positive response to you as a *person*. He or she could give you *honest* positive feedback. This type of response can help free you from constantly comparing yourself to other "bodies" and from trying to emulate a plastic standard of beauty. This doesn't mean that your therapist should discourage you from changing your body into a healthier one. (For example, if you are overweight, some positive reactions from your therapist could help you start to lose weight.)

Most women hate their bodies. They feel that their bodies are separated from the rest of their being. This alienation is a very painful thing. It limits a woman's capacity to act as a whole human being, to move, to make love. It is something that a good therapist will not reinforce, but will help you struggle against.

ON HAVING ORGASMS

Your therapist may have in mind a definite model for what an orgasm is and how or where you should experience it. Women's orgasms have been described *ad nauseum* by men for decades—in novels, in marriage manuals, in psychology textbooks. While men seem to know just what an orgasm should be, women are often confused and report a tremendous variety of experiences—when they report at all.

We found from talking among ourselves and our friends that each of us had our own definite idea of what an orgasm felt like, but no one description could cover everybody's experience. It was even hard for some of us to generalize about ourselves because of the variety we experienced from one time to another.

Recollection of Orgasms

Some of the variety on orgasms reflected in the following phrases may result from the difficulty of finding words for the inexpressible; but they also cover a genuine difference in aspects of orgasm like length, intensity, where it's felt, how it's achieved.

Orgasms feel like: an explosion, a shiver, a sudden flash in the dark, velvet waves, spasms of muscles all over, a labor contraction, a pinpoint of sensation gone almost before it comes, a long screech that seems like it won't ever stop, a great clapping of muscles, a series of instant flashes, ripply, one giant and a lot of remembering flashes, a bursting rainbow of colors, of whiteness, a constant pitch of excitement merging right into orgasm, something sharply different from anything before. They can be gentle, painful, gradual, instantaneous, sharp, sweet, spontaneous, or the result of a lot of work. They can leave you feeling exhausted, unmoving, almost dead, they can leave your body a fiery nerve—one light touch and you're off again, or they can satisfy you for days or leave you ready for more right away.

Where we feel orgasms: uterus, clitoris, vagina, all over, breasts, ears, from the center of the body flowing out to the fingertips, localized, spread all over, deep inside or on the surface.

When we have orgasms: with men, with women, alone— before the lover's, after the lover's, at the same time as the lover's, while masturbating, during intercourse, not during intercourse, never during intercourse, while dreaming or fantasizing. While rocking on the bannister or the arm of the old red couch. They may come with finger or tongue manipulation, in a variety of positions, only one position, with gentle stroking or hard rubbing, with powerful thrusting or gentle moving during intercourse, right away or after a long time, with steady rhythms or broken.

But many sex manuals, therapists, women, and men often have a single model for what women's orgasm should be like, when they should come, and where they should be felt. Any woman who doesn't measure up to this standard too often thinks of herself or is thought to be inadequate, abnormal, maybe even "frigid" or cold. Many women, accepting this model, don't trust their own experience and get caught in a trap of self-doubt—do I have "real" orgasms? The earth doesn't move, I don't see explosions of stars, I don't feel anything happen in my vagina, I never come during intercourse —am I a "real" woman? And behind the silent fear is that haunting line from all the manuals and women's magazines— *If you've ever had an orgasm, you know it.* If you don't know, you haven't had it. But how can any single idea of orgasm be right when even our small group couldn't come up with one definition that included all of us, much less the experiences of all women?

It's not only the idea that all orgasms are the same that can make it rough on you. This single model for orgasms is male- (or penis-) centered. It's based on male experience. It assumes that a woman's orgasm must be some version of a man's. This use of male experience as a norm for female sexuality is evident in Freud's description of masturbation:

> If during the phallic phase [a young girl] attempts to get pleasure like a boy by the manual stimulation of her genitals, it often happens that she fails to obtain sufficient gratification and extends her judgment of inferiority from her stunted penis to her whole self.[11]

Women are urged in sex manuals, women's magazines, and novels to learn to experience their ultimate climax at the same time as the man's. But such an aim assumes that women's orgasms are like a man's, that women come only once in one big rush as the result of forceful thrust. How are multiple orgasms supposed to fit into this scheme? What about the woman whose orgasms never come during intercourse? What about the woman who makes love only with other women? Are the orgasms of these women inferior to those of the rare woman who has managed to adjust her rhythm to the man's?

We have been told that we should not equate therapists' ideas about sexuality with the prejudices and ignorance of the general culture or with the writers of popular sex manuals. Therapists are supposedly at the forefront of the move to break down sexual inhibitions. Historically, this has certainly been true. In nineteenth-century Europe and America, sexual feelings in women were considered abnormal and dangerous for a woman's mental health. But at the end of the Victorian era, Freud made a great contribution by insisting that the expression of sexual desire was natural, healthy, and important for both men and women. As a legacy from the early days of Freud's psychoanalysis, therapists often do encourage the release and blossoming of sexuality in women. But when they do so and at the same time remain ignorant about female sexuality, they tend to see the *male* sexual experience as the model for *human* sexuality; in this case women are not likely to find sexual fulfillment through such therapy.

The controversy over vaginal versus clitoral orgasms (started by Freud and still continuing as a hot subject today) supports our suspicion that many therapists still see women's sexual experience through male eyes. According to the two-orgasm theory, the model for the ideal woman goes something like this—a young girl masturbating gets her orgasms by manipulating her clitoris with her finger—and she feels her orgasm in the clitoris. The mature woman learns to have a "superior" vaginal orgasm from the friction of the penis. It is supposed to be this orgasm (achieved only via a man) that is profound, earthshaking, and a sign of full womanhood—probably because it is first of all a sign of the virility of the male.

Freud wrote:

> ... all their [little girls'] masturbatory acts are carried out on this penis-equivalent, and ... the truly feminine vagina is still undiscovered by both sexes ... in the phallic phase the clitoris is the leading erotogenic zone. But it is not, of course, going to remain so. With the change to femininity the clitoris should wholly or in part hand over its sensitivity, and at the same time its importance, to the vagina.[12]

In Lois Gould's *Such Good Friends*, the female protagonist muses:

> I wonder if he's sorry he told me all that crap about two kinds of female orgasm. "The clitoral, which of course you've experienced, is very nice," he said, "but it's nothing compared to the deep fulfillment of the *vaginal*. Only the male can give that." You were a little nutsy yourself about that Doctor, but it only hung me up another seven or eight years, until they proved there was only one kind of female orgasm after all and we could stop torturing ourselves about not getting Brand X. That's right, ladies, no cock can do any more for you than you can do with a finger or tongue or this handy cordless plastic vibrator ($4.95, batteries extra; available in ivory, or pink or heaven blue).[13]

The assumption that women have two kinds of orgasms and the belief that the superior orgasm is dependent on male penetration are both male-oriented notions of female sexuality. First of all, these attitudes imply that orgasms stimulated by masturbation, during "foreplay" and "afterplay," or through lesbian sexual experiences, are inferior. Secondly, they suggest indirectly that male sexual needs are primary, and that a woman fulfills herself sexually by adjusting what arouses her to what pleases her male partner.

Alexander Lowen, a psychotherapist whose books sell very widely, wrote in *Love and Orgasm* about women: "The problem of orgastic potency in a woman is complicated by the fact that some women are capable of experiencing a sexual climax through clitoral stimulation. ... Most men, however, feel that the need to bring a woman to climax through clitoral stimulation is a burden." Lowen goes on to explain that if the man must do this when he is ready to penetrate, this delay "imposes a restraint upon his natural desire for closeness and intimacy." Clitoral stimulation during intercourse "distracts" the man and "greatly interferes with the pelvic movements upon which his own feeling of satisfaction depends." Clitoral stimulation after intercourse is "burdensome since it prevents him from enjoying the relaxation and peace" that orgasm brings. After stating that most men he has spoken to who have used clitoral stimulation "resented" the need to do so, Lowen continues with his own recommendation: "I do not mean to condemn the practice of clitoral stimulation if a woman finds that this is the way she can obtain sexual release. . . . However, I advise my patients against this practice since it focuses feelings on the clitoris and prevents the vaginal response. It is not a fully satisfactory experience and cannot be considered the equivalent of a vaginal orgasm." Elsewhere in his book, Lowen speaks of women's "right to sexual fulfillment" and the need for women to "speak for themselves" about their sexual needs. But the generosity of his intention is undercut by his belief in the two-orgasm theory and the superiority of the orgasm that is not perceived as a burden to or does not interfere with male sexual needs.[14]

Lowen's perpetuation of the belief in two kinds of orgasms was published just before Masters' and Johnson's tremendously important research on female sexuality, *Human Sexual Response* (1966), became widely publicized. It is difficult to accurately assess the influence of this new research on those who had held such fundamental assumptions about female sexuality as the two-orgasm theory or the primacy of male needs. But by now, the Masters and Johnson research contradicting such assumptions is highly respected and widely accepted.

Briefly, here is what Masters and Johnson have argued on the basis of their observation (with electronic devices) of the physiology of female arousal and orgasm. They found absolutely no basis for the belief in two separate orgasms. They said the woman's orgasm "happens" in the muscles that form the "floor" of the whole genital area (these muscles in the perineum are the same ones you would use to hold back urine); an orgasm is the contraction (or contractions) of these muscles. But it is the stimulation of the clitoris, not the vagina, which can bring about these contractions or orgasms. The vagina itself, Masters and Johnson pointed out, has very sparse nerve endings. Therefore, if all stimulation is localized to the vagina, the woman has little chance of becoming aroused. Orgasm occurs far more rapidly if the clitoris is either directly or indirectly stimulated during love-making, they point out.[15]

However, it is not necessary to believe that measuring women's physiological responses with electrodes tells us all we need to know about the total psychological and physical experience of women's sexuality. We believe that no one should tell you what kind of orgasm to have—where you should feel it; whether you should do it with men, women, or by yourself; whether you can or cannot have orgasms during intercourse. We think whatever gives you pleasure, whatever leaves you with a feeling of warmth and satisfaction instead of tension and loneliness, is OK. And if your therapist wants to talk about your orgasms, ask yourself if he or she makes any assumptions about what you *should* experience. Rather than measuring yourself against these or any other standards, trust your own sensations and feelings. Trust your own body —it's beautiful.

ON NOT HAVING ORGASMS

I just made love with a man and as usual, I didn't have an orgasm. He says, immediately after, "Did you come?" I think, "He's asking me if I liked it, if I like him; he's asking me if my body is responding in the way everyone says it's supposed to, if I'm normal, if making love for me is all it's supposed to be, if I am a real woman."
I answer "Yes."

If you're not having orgasms you may be afraid you're "frigid"; this is a fear that may send you to a therapist. One therapist told us that a great majority of the women who came to her are afraid they are "frigid" and will never have satisfying sexual relationships. Many women face this dilemma, and face it alone—because women seldom talk to each other about their sexual experiences.

We believe that many therapists would probably reinforce your fears of "frigidity." Therapists who have had a great deal of psychoanalytical training may start asking you questions about your childhood relationship to your father; or if they are the kind of therapists who haven't questioned the sexual socialization of women, they are likely to assume you are not a warm, responsive, "real" woman. In short, therapists are likely to blame you or your early childhood instead of seeing the source of your problem elsewhere. It is questionable whether the concept of "frigidity" has any validity at all; therapists' use of this category has been very destructive to women. First of all, the word "frigid" implies, subtly if not directly, that if you're not having orgasms, it's your own fault. "Frigidity" is *your* condition, *your* quality, *your* failure. And most women who are not having orgasms feel overwhelmingly guilty and inadequate. Your therapist will most likely reinforce these feelings. Also, "frigidity" in its common usage is often a static term implying permanence—a woman who's been told that she's "frigid" may literally *freeze* with the fear she'll always remain so, a self-fulfilling prophecy.

Some of the research done by other sexologists raises further questions about whom the word "frigid" can be applied to. In her article "The Phallacy of Our Sexual Norm," Karen Rotkin discusses a variety of studies that claim that two-thirds to three-fourths of all women masturbate. They are cited as reaching orgasm about 95 percent of the time, a higher rate of orgasm than women experience in any other kind of sexual activity.[16] Women who seldom, if ever, have orgasms during intercourse are often labeled "frigid" by themselves and their doctors. But many of these women are not "frigid" at all. They have a great capacity for orgasm from direct clitoral stimulation, but they are simply not aroused to have orgasms by friction from intercourse. Thus "frigidity" is frequently understood in phallocentric terms—you're "frigid" if you don't have an orgasm as the direct result of a man's penis inside you.

Another problem with the word "frigid" is raised by Masters and Johnson research discrediting the two-orgasm theory. Many therapists who still distinguish between vaginal and clitoral orgasms would call a woman who said she had only clitoral orgasms "frigid" or immature. This kind of therapist would certainly say that an orgasm reached during lesbian love-making, masturbation, or the "sexual play" before or after intercourse, is typical of a woman whose sexual development has been "arrested." Such a concept of "frigidity"—based as it is on the two-orgasm theory—has clearly been outdated by the Masters and Johnson research. The many women who do not have an orgasm when a penis is in the vagina are not "frigid"—they are not having an orgasm because the clitoris is not being aroused by any friction. There can be lots of reasons why the friction of intercourse doesn't affect the clitoris. The location of the clitoris and the shaft of the clitoris is different for every woman. Women whose clitoris is closer to the vaginal entrance are more likely to have orgasms during intercourse. The positions used in intercourse can also greatly change the degree of excitement —though there is certainly no one position that will give pleasure to all women.

A woman in her thirties told us:

While I was pregnant and later tired from caring for three infants and toddlers at all hours of the day and night, I didn't have much interest in sex. I avoided it and seldom received much satisfaction from it. But when the children were not so demanding, I really felt a great desire for sexual expression—I wanted suddenly an active and satisfying sexual relationship with my husband. It was practically impossible for us to talk out loud about our sexual problems. But silently, we kept experimenting and suddenly we came upon a position that worked like a miracle for me. I felt excitement and orgasms that I had never had before. I now have a deep confidence and joy in myself as a sexual human being. But if we make love in the tradi-

*tional way—the man on top—I don't feel anything again. In our
special position, there's no problem.*

From discussions among ourselves, with our friends, and
from what a woman therapist told us, it appears that a great
number of women who regularly have orgasms at some point
during love-making never have them during intercourse (when
the penis is in the vagina). Shere Hite's report based on her
nationwide survey of women's sexuality showed that *"only
approximately 30 percent of the women in this study could
orgasm regularly from intercourse."*[17] Obviously the women
in the remaining 70 percent are not "frigid," though a therapist might consider them so; and given the emphasis on intercourse in this culture, those women themselves might feel
inadequate.

If the term "frigid" can have any valid meaning at all,
it should be purely physiological, referring only to a woman
whose clitoris or perineal muscles do not function. But un-
fortunately, the common use of the word "frigid" implies a
whole range of psychological qualities instead of simply physical ones. By calling a woman "frigid," a therapist may be
assuming and indirectly suggesting that she is cold, unloving,
selfish, incapable of giving or receiving love. Implicitly, a
male therapist may wonder how any "real" woman could
resist arousal while she is in bed with a man. He may hold out
the possibility of a "cure" by suggesting that she learn to be
a fully responsive, warm, supportive woman.

What can you do if you're not having orgasms? Rather
than jumping to the conclusion that you're "frigid," you
should consider some of the possible reasons for your difficulty. To begin with, women generally have very little knowledge about their bodies—what their sexual organs are, how
they're related, what an orgasm is, what excites them sexually. One woman told us, "I didn't even know I had a clitoris
until I was 27. I just always thought that men had penises
and women had vaginas." Such ignorance is made worse by
the fact that most discussions of female sexuality assume

that the woman's experience is some minor version or else the completely passive product of the man's energetic virtuosity —as in the following passage:

> He took her to the bedroom and undressed her slowly, he made love to her beautifully. Nothing frantic, nothing rushed. He caressed her body as though there were nothing more important in the world. He took her to the edge of ecstasy and back again, keeping her hovering, sure of every move he made. Her breasts grew under his touch, swelling, becoming even larger and firmer. She floated on a suspended plane, a complete captive to his hands and body. He had amazing control, stopping at just the right moment. When it did happen it was only because he wanted it to, and they came in complete unison. She had never experienced *that* before, and she clung to him, words tumbling out of her mouth about how much she loved him. Afterwards they lay and smoked and talked. "You're wonderful," he said. "You're a clever woman making me wait until after we were married!"[18]

Because women are ignorant of their own sexuality, they often don't know what kind of movements, pressures, and positions are most likely to bring on an orgasm or series of orgasms. This ignorance, or the belief that they must be passive, is a greater cause of not having orgasms than "frigidity."

Even if a woman knows what she likes, she's often afraid of telling her lover what to do during love-making. She may fear that any suggestion on her part will be taken as criticism that might hurt her lover. As we said earlier, the medical experts of the nineteenth century actually believed and taught that "normal" women had no sexual feelings at all. Sex was a woman's duty—something to be endured by her for the sake of the husband and procreation. When a woman felt aroused or had an orgasm, she often felt guilty, as if sexual passion proved that she was not a "lady." One good thing Freud and the psychologists who followed him did was to recognize that women *do* have a sexual nature and should try to develop it naturally. For at least twenty years, sex manuals have told couples how to bring that difficult woman to climax.

But something subtle has happened—the woman is still

seen as the passive, receptive one (seldom the initiator) whose body is worked on by her skillful, virile lover. Her orgasm has become first of all proof of her lover's manhood and only secondarily a pleasure for *her*. So if you are not having orgasms, you may be caught in a vicious circle. To ask your lover to change his style, his rhythms, his timing, and so forth is to tell him he has been no good for you, that he is a lousy lover. Here you are faced with the familiar female crunch—will you be supportive, keeping your unhappiness or your faked orgasms to yourself? Or will you recognize your own needs? The culture gives all the approval to the first solution and not the second. And to make this worse, your tension and worry about all these things and what you might see as your failure may make you so up-tight that you won't be able to let yourself "go" with your sensations. You may begin to dread sex. And if you tell your therapist you avoid sex, make excuses, etc., chances are the he or she will start asking you about your father, your initial sexual encounters, your fantasies, your attitude toward men—all of which will probably increase your sense of inadequacy.

The question you must ask yourself is whether you can break out of this circle by breaking the silence. Can you and your lover work *together* toward mutual satisfaction? You will probably have to be the one to initiate change. And since we don't think many therapists are ahead of the rest of society in understanding women's sexuality—if anything, their training is likely to put them behind—we don't think you'll get much support or encouragement from your therapist.

The difficulty two people have in communicating about sex is immense. But if we women are ever to put behind us the lonely and unfulfilling experience of faking orgasms, we will have to break the wall of silence, start believing that our own pleasure is as important as that of our lover's, and start asking for some experimentation with different positions, rhythms, movements, types of stimulation. The courage to start asking will have to be ours.

The picture we have painted of the kind of "help" you are likely to get for sexual problems may seem quite bleak. And if you have little chance of seeing a nontraditional therapist for geographic or economic reasons, this picture is probably fairly accurate. But new research on female sexuality is gradually being absorbed by many therapists. Masters and Johnson in particular are having some concrete impact on therapists. For a high tuition, they train sex therapists in their method of working with people who have sexual problems. Other nontraditional therapists and feminist therapists are using the Masters and Johnson research to develop new ways of helping women. Times and attitudes in the culture at large have changed since 1968 or so—just how much still remains to be seen. But training can help reverse the kinds of attitudes about female sexuality we have grown up with.

Many large cities have sex clinics where therapists who don't consciously hold traditional views on female sexuality tend to concentrate. If you live in a big city, look for such clinics; you may find the help you need. But evaluate these therapists carefully, just as you need to do for other aspects of therapy.

Smaller cities or towns are much less likely to have whole clinics of therapists who openly share nontraditional or feminist attitudes toward therapy, although there are of course scattered individual therapists who have questioned the accepted sexual norms of society. And considering how little real help is available for women with sexual problems, we realize that the number of women going to sex clinics is very small compared to the numbers of women who turn to their doctors and ministers, priests and rabbis for advice.

You may sense that our discussion of therapy and female sexuality vacillates between the belief that therapy as it is today offers minimal help to women and the hope that therapy may become an avenue to more complete sexual fulfillment for some women. This seeming contradiction emerges out of the firm conviction that women's sexual problems, like sex-role problems, *must be placed in their social context.* To be understood, the various individual problems of women's sexuality must be analyzed in terms of how each woman has responded to the dominant cultural attitudes toward sexuality. We believe that the potential of the therapeutic process to help women with sexual problems depends greatly on how the therapist responds to the challenges of feminism to re-think general cultural perspectives on women's sexuality.

Feminist scholars and activists have argued that women's sexual expression has been repressed, controlled, and defined in terms of men and male needs in a variety of ways depending on the culture and historical period. Cliterodectomy (operation to remove parts of the perineal area), purdah (complete seclusion of women to women's quarters in the home), absolute monogamy (for women), and footbinding are some of the more extreme forms of this repression. But women's sexuality has also been controlled in some of the following ways, many of which will be familiar to you: common attitudes that women are sexually passive while men are sexual initiators; cultural divisions of women into "good girls" (sexually chaste) and "bad girls" (whores), ladies and prostitutes; the double sexual standards for men and women; the reduction of women to sex objects—especially in the media, where erotic images of women are used to sell products and excite male fantasy; sadistic and psychotic violence committed against women; women's fear of beatings or rape as restrictive of free movement; the belief that women cause and enjoy rape; competition fostered among women to be the most "beautiful," according to some arbitrary standard; the condemnation of lesbian sexuality as unnatural, sick, and incomplete; the legal statutes which give husbands the right to coerce their wives to have sex; the link often made between sexual expression and procreation for women, especially for women whose religion or culture prohibits or discourages birth control; the limitations placed on a woman's right to control her body—if and when she will conceive, give birth or be sterilized; and so forth.[19]

Placed within the context of these general issues, your individual difficulties with your sexuality have some chance of resolution. Some women have begun to free themselves of such cultural restrictions through sharing feelings, ideas, and experiences with supportive women and men who are also working to change. And some women have found therapists with whom they can explore ways to transcend the traditional definitions of women's sexuality.

FOOTNOTES

[1]James Hemming, *Problems in Adolescent Girls* (London: Heinemann, 1950), pp. 93-94. See Germaine Greer's discussion of Hemming and the adolescent girl's fear of being unattractive in *The Female Eunuch* (New York: Bantam Books, 1970), p. 85.

[2]Sigmund Freud, "Femininity," in *New Introductory Lectures*, trans. James Strachey (New York: W. W. Norton, 1964), pp. 126, 132.

[3]Greer, *The Female Eunuch*, p. 45.

[4]Phyllis Chesler, *Women and Madness* (New York: Doubleday, 1972), p. 225. Excerpts from *Women and Madness* by Phyllis Chesler. Copyright © 1972 by Phyllis Chesler. Reprinted by permission of Doubleday & Company, Inc. and Penguin Books Ltd.

[5]Ibid., p. 169.

[6]William H. Grier and Price M. Cobbs, *Black Rage* (New York: Bantam Books, 1968), pp. 46-62.

[7]Ibid., p. 33.

[8]Ibid., p. 40.

[9]Ibid. Black women writers have explored the impact of white standards of beauty with a greater understanding of how body image relates to all the other aspirations Black women have. See especially Toni Morrison, *The Bluest Eye* (New York: Pocket Books, 1970) and Alice Walker, *Meridian* (New York: Pocket Books, 1976).

[10]Ibid., pp. 43-44.

[11]Sigmund Freud, *An Outline of Psychoanalysis*, trans. James Strachey (New York: Norton, 1949), p. 97.

[12]Freud, "Femininity," p. 118.

[13]Lois Gould, *Such Good Friends* (New York: Random House, 1970), p. 95.

[14]Alexander Lowen, *Love and Orgasm* (New York: Macmillan, 1965), pp. 215, 216-17.

[15]William H. Masters and Virginia E. Johnson, *Human Sexual Response* (Boston: Little, Brown and Co., 1966), pp. 65-67, 77-78, 129. See especially Chapter 5, "The Clitoris," and Chapter 9, "The Female Orgasm."

[16]Karen F. Rotkin, "The Phallacy of Our Sexual Norm," *Rough Times*, 3, no. 1 (September 1972), 20–21. This excellent article was a great help to us in writing this section. *Rough Times* was first called *The Radical Therapist* and is now called *State and Mind*.

[17]Shere Hite, *The Hite Report: A Nationwide Study of Female Sexuality* (New York: Dell, 1976), p. 134. The women in Hite's study were not chosen on the basis of a random sample; consequently, this percentage might or might not hold true for the general population of women.

[18]Jackie Collins, *The World Is Full of Married Men* (Cleveland, Ohio: World Publishing Co., 1969), pp. 152–53. See also Greer's analysis of the sexual androcentrism evident in Collins' book, *The Female Eunuch*, p. 39.

[19]For some references to feminist books and articles on female sexuality, see the bibliography at the end of the book.

Psychological Theory and the Therapist

As you look for a therapist, you may wonder what all the different titles mean and what they might reflect about the training and methods of each therapist. The number of years of training and the type of program can vary greatly.

If your therapist calls him/herself a *psychiatrist*, then you know automatically that he/she has an M.D. degree plus three or four years of "resident" training in psychotherapy. This residency involves classroom study of psychology and at least one year of doing therapy under supervision. There is no single training program for psychiatrists—each school varies in requirements, types of courses offered, and probably emphasis. You can be quite certain, however, that a psychiatrist has had to study "classical" psychology—the theories of Freud, Jung, Erikson, the neo-Freudians, Rollo May, and so forth. Some people feel that because psychiatrists have had this classical background, they are more likely to be traditional in method and outlook. One thing is certain: a psychiatrist is an M.D. as well and can therefore prescribe drugs as a part of your treatment.

If your therapist is called a *psychoanalyst*, you can be certain his or her training in Freudian theory has been extensive. "Psychoanalysis" was the name Freud chose to call his school of psychology; any therapist who uses this term associates with a Freudian or neo-Freudian perspective. Freud and the early psychoanalysts were all M.D.'s as well, and for the most part, this is still true. In this kind of therapy, you can expect a basic framework of Freudian ideas, which usually carries with it an assumption that therapy will be long-term (several years at least) and will focus on dream analysis and reconstruction of your early childhood.

An *analytical psychologist* has gone through another type of "classical" training that focuses heavily on dream analysis. "Analytical psychology" was Carl Jung's name for his school. Jung was first a disciple of Freud, then something of an enemy, and he used this title in the early days of psychoanalysis to distinguish his approach from Freud's.

If your therapist is called a *psychologist*, he/she most likely has a Ph.D. degree in clinical psychology (and *no* M.D.). Ph.D. programs differ all over the country: various ones may have developed reputations for being "behaviorist," "existentialist," "eclectic" (teaching all approaches), etc. Your therapist's particular training is likely to depend on which school he or she attended. Clinical psychology programs require some kind of supervised therapy as well as classroom study of psychological theory and method. Psychologists cannot prescribe drugs, but they can make arrangements with a psychiatrist who will write the prescription for them.

There are many therapists without M.D.'s or Ph.D.'s— their backgrounds rest on a wide variety of programs. *Social workers* who do therapy may have been through a MSW (Masters in Social Work) program. In New York graduate schools, this degree takes two years of course work and supervised field work. *Psychiatric nurses* often do residency work right along with the psychiatry residents. There are also a number of *intern programs* which require a fairly short period of intensive study and on-the-job training. One such program in Chicago involved about a semester's study, and guaranteed each student a job as a therapist at the end of the training. Each week the interns were introduced to a new set of psychological theories and techniques (transactional analysis, bioenergetics, gestalt therapy, family therapy, etc.); the whole group met as a therapy group itself, and toward the end each intern was placed in an out-patient facility or mental hospital to *assist* in therapy situations.

Certainly this kind of apprenticeship training and social work program does not offer the kind of extensive "classical" training available to a psychoanalyst, psychiatrist, or even a psychologist. This does not necessarily mean, however, that the therapist with less intensive training will be less likely to label and "treat" you in traditional ways. Freudian tenets can be applied as dogmatically by someone with only a smattering of knowledge as by a person who has had years of study. You will have to evaluate for yourself what the impact of any particular training has been on your therapist.

Women counseling other women—*feminist lay counseling* —is another kind of therapy that is mushrooming in parts of the country where the women's movement is strong. Often working with the advice and help of other women with degrees in psychology, psychiatry, social work, etc., women with no specialized psychiatric training offer counsel to women who seek nontraditional therapy. Their expertise is based perhaps on an orientation training for new counselors, discussions with other women counselors, and most of all a sensitivity to the psychological difficulties of growing up female in a society that limits women and discriminates institutionally and economically against them.

In your evaluation of the impact training has had on your therapist, it will be helpful for you to know about some of the major theories about women that are part of most therapists' training. Your therapist may or may not identify with one particular school. In smaller communities, therapists may deny any theoretical association and call themselves "eclectic"; in large cities, there are always therapists willing to label themselves. You can find Freudians, Jungians, feminist therapists, gestalt therapists, behaviorists, transactional analysts—the list is endless. But whatever the label, psychological theories about women may have been part of a therapist's training and may have reinforced certain attitudes he/she has about women. We are not suggesting that you judge the quality of a therapist by his or her label. A good therapist will be good despite the biases of any theories, and a sexist therapist will be sexist with *or* without them. Still, we think you should know something about the psychological theories involved in your therapist's training, and how this affects the assumptions he/she makes about you as a woman. This can have a great effect on how he or she interprets the things you talk about.

THE FREUDIAN PSYCHOANALYST

Of psychoanalysis, Germaine Greer wrote: "Freud is the father of psychoanalysis. It had no mother."[1] And Freud himself began his lecture on "Femininity" with an affirmation of his empirical objectivity:

> I can say two things to recommend it ["today's lecture"]. *It brings forward nothing but observed facts* [italics added], almost without speculative additions, and it deals with a subject which has a claim on your interest second almost to no other. Throughout history people have knocked their heads against the riddle of the nature of femininity. . . . Nor will *you* have escaped worrying over this problem— those of you who are men; to those of you who are women this will not apply—you are yourselves the problem.[2]

Freud didn't write much about women, but the few essays he wrote forced women into the masculine model, which is based above all on the happy possession of the penis. His belief that a woman's innately inferior anatomy determines her destiny—that her life is either a hopeless quest for the missing penis or a passive submission to her subordinate role before men—has had a tremendous impact on all kinds of therapists. Psychoanalysts are by definition Freudian or neo-Freudian, and approximately one-tenth of the psychiatrists in the American Psychiatric Association call themselves Freudians. And other psychiatrists, psychologists, and social workers—even when they negate or ridicule parts of Freud's theories—have themselves gone through a training program permeated with Freudian myths about women.

The therapist influenced by Freud—and even the Freudian analyst—might never talk to you about your anatomy, but he or she will have a model of female development in mind into which you will be put no matter what you say. As he or she sees it, your problems all go back to your early childhood —to the happy days you spent before you discovered you didn't have a penis and to the traumatic adjustment you had to make after the fateful day when you first noticed that little boys have, in Freud's words, "far superior equipment." Before this discovery, "a little girl is a little man," Freud says —she is aggressive, intelligent, active, and lively, all qualities Freud assigns to "masculinity." And she has almost as much pleasure in manipulating her clitoris—which Freud calls a woman's "stunted penis"—as a little boy has in manipulating his penis. The "turning point" in a girl's growth comes with "the discovery that she is castrated," when she first sees what she could have gotten in the way of genitals if her luck had been better. (Freud doesn't say the little girl *thinks* she's castrated and inferior; he says she *is* castrated and her sexual apparatus *is* innately inferior and "defective.")[3]

The kind of woman the little girl becomes is determined by her reaction to this physiological discovery. The classical Freudian analyst will put you into one of three categories. Category 1: you never got over the trauma of castration and thereby became a totally inhibited, neurotic woman who can't function in the real world. Category 2: as a little girl you refused to accept the fact you could never have a penis, with the result that your basic drives as an adult woman are shaped by this hidden desire to be a man. In this case you are labeled a "masculine woman," and your desire for independence and a job, your interest in intellectual, scientific, or mechanical matters, your personal strength and inability to play a submissive or "normal feminine" role are all aspects of your "masculinity complex." In this role your self-assertions are "aggressive" (a negative quality in a woman) and originate in your unconscious wish for a penis. So *whatever* you seek or do or say outside the home is regarded by the Freudian analyst as "sublimations" of penis envy.

In Category 2, as a "masculine woman," you may be able to make it in the world of men, but your relationships—especially your love relationships—with men will rarely be successful. The extreme form of the "masculine woman" is the lesbian, whose penis envy, Freudians say, is carried to the point of sickness. If you have a husband, the marriage will be a tense one because your "masculine" qualities will not be supportive —their effect will be "castrating" and destructive to men. In practice, the term "masculine woman" is often just a euphemism for "castrating bitch." And your desire for time of your own demonstrates your inability to fulfill the role of a sacrificing mother—*you*, not your husband, nor your family situation, nor your social environment—will be blamed for your children's problems or the failure of your marriage. Freud believed that most women seek therapy because of an unresolved penis envy. He believed that most women who are dissatisfied with their lives are unhappy because of personal inadequacy and "arrested" feminine development, rather than because of any injustices in society. Even women psychoanalysts were not exempt from Freud's categorization:

> Thus we shall not be so very surprised if a woman analyst who has not been sufficiently convinced of the intensity of her own desire for a penis also fails to assign an adequate importance to that factor in her patients.[4]

Category 3: your third possible response to your discovery of "castration" takes you on the route to what Freudians call "normal femininity." Unlike the "masculine woman," whose development is considered to be arrested in the "masculine phase," you adjust yourself to your anatomical inferiority, and your former activity and assertiveness turns to passivity. You start playing with dolls as preparation for the baby you will have someday. Your future husband and your child—especially a male child—will give you vicariously the "longed-for penis" that you lack. As Freud wrote:

> The feminine situation is only established, however, if the wish for a penis is replaced by one for a baby . . . quite especially so if the baby is a little boy who brings the longed-for penis with him.[5]

Qualities of the normal "feminine woman" will be qualities that are considered unhealthy in a man—masochism (you exult in sacrificing yourself for others); passivity (you give up your own ideas and desires and become submissive to men); narcissism (you are vain about your appearance as an understandable overcompensation for your inferiority). Your dedication to family means that you lack the strong superego men have—that is, you have few ties and make no contributions to culture, tradition, and civilization. And finally, with your sister the "masculine woman," you have "little sense of justice" as a result of the "predominance of envy" (penis envy) in your "mental life."[6]

Many therapists who *don't* want to concentrate on your children—even those who might say that Freud's ideas about the castration complex are a lot of nonsense—may still knowingly or unknowingly use these categories of the "masculine" and "feminine" woman. Of all Freud's theories, the one that is most likely to survive in the therapist's office is the assumption that the woman who wants a life of her own has no chance of a happy life with a man, with children, or with other women. According to most therapists, to be "feminine," you must give up any idea of a separate world of productive work outside the home; and to be a "masculine woman," you must give up any idea of a family.

It was just this crunch, with its denial of a full humanity —work and love—that drove Sylvia Plath's hero Esther Greenwood in *The Bell Jar* to withdrawal, self-hate, and attempted suicide. Esther didn't want the cold, sexless life of the career woman Jay Cee; nor did she want the vegetating content of the suburban breeder Dodo Conway (woman as mother) or the selfish, workless, and cynical life of the sexy Doreen (woman as siren). When her boyfriend asked her if she would like to be "Mrs. Buddy Willard," doctor's wife, she said she didn't want to have to choose either a life in the country or a life in the city. She wanted both. Buddy's response was the Freudian one—he accused Esther of having the "perfect neurotic set-up." The traditional psychiatrist Esther first saw treated her neurosis with electroshock therapy and enthusiastic comments about the WACS stationed at Esther's college during the war. Result: attempted suicide. The therapist who helped Esther was a warm, loving, supportive woman who was also a "Dr."—maintaining that very combination of work and love that Esther wanted for herself.[7]

If you, like Esther, struggle against this enforced choice between being the "feminine woman" or the "masculine woman," your therapist may point the finger of blame at *you*, and not at the choice he or she or your family or the culture at large is forcing you to make. Your therapist just may start you on a guilt trip from which you'll never return.

Problems that have to do with marriage, love relationships, desires and uncertainties about our own capabilities, and frustrations about jobs are the problems we most often bring to therapists. These are exactly the areas Freudians have so many preconceptions about; they are the areas that are affected most by their constricting categorizations. You should try to examine your therapist's assumptions about women very carefully in order to avoid being placed into one of these limiting roles.

Some neo-Freudians, as well as psychoanalysts, have

also created theoretical models of female psychology based ultimately on female anatomy. Erik Erikson, for example, argued that little girls build houses out of blocks and little boys build towers as a reflection both of their physiology (womb and penis) and future destiny (mothers and builders):

> Woman's fulfillment rests on the fact that "somatic" design harbors an "inner space" [womb] destined to bear the offspring of chosen men, and with it, a biological, psychological, and ethical commitment to take care of human infancy.[8]

And Joseph Rheingold, a Harvard psychiatrist, wrote:

> Woman is nurturance.... Anatomy decrees the life of a woman.... When women grow up without dread of their biological functions and without subversion by feminist doctrine, and therefore enter upon motherhood with a sense of fulfillment and altruistic sentiment, we shall attain the goal of a good life and a secure world in which to live it.[9]

THE JUNGIAN ANALYTICAL PSYCHOLOGIST

C. G. Jung was more interested in spirit than Freud, and he rejected the way Freud reduced human desires to sex and physiology. But his theories about women can be as devastating as Freud's. Where Freud said a woman's anatomy determined her destiny, Jung gave mystical and spiritual reasons why women were and should be passive, submissive, emotional, and subjective.

Jungian theories on women have proved attractive to women because Jung never wrote about woman as an inferior or castrated version of man, as Freud did. Jung and Jungians after him believed in inherent feminine and masculine qualities that were opposite and complementary. A Jungian would see you as the modern incarnation of the Great Earth Mother in your positive fulfillment and as a devouring, castrating witch or Medusa in your demonic, man-engulfing forms (e.g., the overprotective mother). Jungians view the unconscious as predominantly feminine, and their descriptions of the unconscious often reflect this dual imagery of extremes. For example, Erich Neumann, a Jungian disciple, wrote:

> The overwhelming might of the unconscious, i.e., the devouring, destructive aspect under which it may manifest itself, is seen figuratively as the evil mother, whether as the bloodstained goddess of death, famine, flood, and the force of instinct, or as the sweetness that lures to destruction. But, as the good mother, she is fullness and abundance; the dispenser of life and happiness, the nutrient earth, the cornucopia of the fruitful womb.[10]

What makes Jungian theory attractive to women is the sense of great importance and mystical fertility you can accept as your Earth-Mother destiny. The hidden danger is that Jung's theories provide a religious and mythical language for the all-too-familiar cultural norms. The future your Jungian analyst would project for you as a "real" woman would of course include a mate and children. Neumann limited the creative sphere for women to their reproductive role:

> The creative energy of woman comes alive in the miracle of birth, by virtue of which she becomes the "Great Mother" and "Earth Goddess."[11]

Unless you desire a mate and children, you are seen as a tiresome, argumentative, "masculine" woman, much as in Freudian theory. Any problems you have will resolve themselves if you will only consent to your spiritual destiny and have a child. Fulfillment comes with the flowering of your "femininity."

M. Esther Harding, another Jungian disciple, placed her defense of traditional "femininity" squarely within the context of her attack on feminism:

> Woman has moved away from the old, well-established, woman's way of conduct and psychological adaptation and finds herself today beset by problems which neither she herself, nor the pioneer women who initiated the movement for women's emancipation foresaw.

These changes have produced for woman an unavoidable inner conflict between the urge to express herself through work, as a man does, and the inner necessity to live in accordance with her own ancient feminine nature. . . . Not infrequently we hear it affirmed that there is no essential difference between men and women, except the biological one. Many women have accepted this standpoint and have themselves done much to foster it. They have been content to be men in petticoats and so have lost touch with the feminine principle within themselves. This is perhaps the main cause of the unhappiness and emotional instability of today. For if woman is out of touch with the feminine principle, which dictates the laws of relatedness, she cannot take the lead in what is after all the feminine realm, that of human relationships.[12]

If you tell your Jungian analyst that to be exclusively a wife and mother leaves you with no individual self-identity, he or she might agree—and then ask you why you *want* an individual identity.

Much like Freud's ideas about women, Jung's theories provided a rationale for the status quo of sex roles: Men and women are innately different, biologically and psychologically. Therefore their roles in life should be complementary, never the same. Women's predominantly "feminine" nature destines her to the domestic sphere of "human relatedness," while man's "masculine" nature gives him the entire public domain and the life of the mind. Jung contrasted the man's world and the woman's world:

Her world is made up of fathers and mothers, brothers and sisters, husbands and children. . . . The man's world is the nation, the state, business concerns, etc. His family is simply a means to an end, one of the foundations of the state, and his wife is not necessarily *the* woman for him (at any rate not as the woman means it when she says "my man"). The general means more to him than the personal; his world consists of a multitude of coordinated factors, whereas her world, outside her husband, terminates in a sort of cosmic mist.[13]

However, Jung's model for the male and female psyches is considerably different from Freud's. Consequently, a Jungian analyst would not be delving into your childhood memories and dreams to uncover various manifestations of penis envy. Jungians are not so much interested in what they called the "personal unconscious," where childhood traumas reside. They interpret many dreams as symbolic messages from the "collective unconscious." Jung believed that therapy could help men and women interpret these images and integrate their meaning into the conscious self in a process called "individuation."

The central image in man's unconscious is the *anima*, the submerged "feminine" self within every man. In dreams, the anima is personified by female images (witches, goddesses, sirens, mothers, sisters, etc.). These representations of women constitute the soul. Individuation for a man involves the integration of the anima, the soul, into his conscious, rational, "masculine" self. The qualities which characterize the anima (emotion, intuition, irrationality, spirituality, vision, etc.) predominate in woman's conscious, "feminine" self. The central image in woman's unconscious is the *animus*, the submerged "masculine" self within every woman. The animus is personified in dreams by male images (wise old men, aggressive heroes, etc.). But Jung's description of the animus does not really parallel and complement his portrait of the anima. The animus is almost always described in negative terms as the aggressive, opinionated, and stubborn inner self that can destroy woman's feminine self. He wrote: "A woman possessed by the animus is always in danger of losing her femininity."[14]

The animus, according to Jung, is the source of a woman's opinions. Woman's "intellect" is not in reality her own; instead woman's ideas are an odd assortment of opinions picked up from the men she listened to while she was a child. As a result, every time a woman argues something, gives an opinion, acts as if she is an intelligent person with ideas, the Jungian can say that it is her animus, her "masculine" self talking. Based on Jung's model, a Jungian therapist can turn all your ideas—anything that isn't subjective emotion—into "opinions," which can be dismissed because they are not yours.

They are merely a residue of the ideas of men you have known. Jung uses this form of dismissal to explain what he sees as women's—particularly *intellectual* women's—stubbornness. Women are hard to reason with, he complained. Men have a terrible time trying to change a woman's mind because they hold on to their opinions with all the irrationality of the unconscious:

> In intellectual women the animus encourages a critical disputatiousness and would-be highbrowism, which, however, consists essentially in harping on some irrelevant weak point and nonsensically making it the main one. ... Without knowing it, such women are solely intent upon exasperating the man and are, in consequence, the more completely at the mercy of the animus. "Unfortunately I am always right," one of these *creatures* [italics added] once confessed to me.[15]

A woman with a pretty face exhibits an adorable petulance when her animus speaks. But plain women who attempt to express an opinion are simply irritating:

> If the woman happens to be pretty, these animus opinions have for the man something rather touching and childlike about them, which makes him adopt a benevolent, fatherly, professional manner. But if the woman does not stir his sentimental side, and competence is expected of her rather than appealing helplessness and stupidity, then her animus opinions irritate the man to death, chiefly because they are based on nothing but opinion for opinion's sake, and "everybody has a right to *his* [italics added] own opinions."[16]

Jung's distaste for the animus seems to be based in part on how uncomfortable it makes life for men. As we would expect, then, individuation for women is not the same process as it is for men. To avoid threatening and exasperating men and to maintain their "femininity," women must learn to "criticize and hold" their "opinions at a distance," essentially to suppress the animus.[17] Women who do not control their animus, "if falsely cultivated, can turn into the worse kind of dogmatist and high-handed pedagogue—a regular 'animus hound,' as one of my woman patients aptly expressed it." The model of individuation Jung posed for women advocates the kind of "feminine" woman who nurtures men:

> Just as a man brings forth his work as a complete creation out of his inner feminine nature, so the inner masculine side of a woman brings forth creative seeds which have the power to fertilize the feminine side of the man.[18]

A Jungian therapist can thus use Jung's concept of the animus to undercut the validity of a woman's expression of ideas, her feelings of anger, and her search for autonomy. This denial of woman's selfhood is represented strikingly in Jung's discussion of the soul:

> Woman has no anima, no soul, but she has an *animus*. The anima has an erotic, emotional character, the animus a rationalizing one. Hence most of what men say about feminine eroticism, and particularly about the emotional life of women, is derived from their own anima projections and distorted accordingly. On the other hand, the astonishing assumptions and fantasies that women make about men come from the activity of the animus, who produces an inexhaustible supply of illogical arguments and false explanations.[19]

From Jung's religious perspective in which he argues that modern Western man is "in search of a soul" destroyed by modern rationalism and technology, the possession of "soul" is the key to a full humanity. Some Jungians claim that Jung really meant by this quote that a woman's "soul" is her animus, but *nowhere* in his description of the qualities of the animus is there even a hint of the positive, religious qualities he associates with the "soul," the anima. It is interesting that Jung so well understood that the "anima" is a projection of male fantasies about women. Why then didn't he apply this concept of projection to his own theories?

BEHAVIORISM

WATCHWORDS TO IDENTIFY A BEHAVIOR MODIFICATION THERAPIST

BEHAVIOR	SYSTEMATIC DESENSITIZATION
STIMULUS	RESPONSE
REINFORCEMENT	ENVIRONMENT

IF YOUR THERAPIST THROWS THESE WORDS AROUND A LOT, IT'S A GOOD BET HE OR SHE IS BEHAVIOR MODIFICATION–ORIENTED.

Behavior modification is founded on the idea that all people deal with one another by reacting to one another's behavior—to things the other person says and does. Behavioral therapists reject the question WHY when examining your problems and look at the events that happen before and after unwanted behavior to figure out what happens in the environment. When what you do is making you or other people (depending on who initiated behavior therapy) miserable, they try to alter the environment so your misery-causing behavior doesn't continue.

Here's an example. I am very anxious all the time and I really can't figure out why. If I go to see a therapist other than a behavioral therapist he or she will probably try to talk to me to find out what experiences in my past caused me to be so nervous and why I still feel threatened. Then this therapist will try to help me stop. A behavioral therapist, however, won't ask me what originally happened to make me so upset. He or she doesn't care, because knowing that won't stop my nervous behavior. Instead, the behaviorist will ask me *when* I am most nervous and *what* usually *happens* after I become nervous. The premise is that there is something in my environment that is *reinforcing* my behavior (making it occur over and over) and *that something* (perhaps it is attention I get from my family and friends) is all that has to be changed. The therapist might deal with the problem by telling my friends to ignore me when I get anxious and give me attention when I'm behaving "normally." This way they'll be reinforcing "normal" behavior. Or this therapist might teach me to relax in situations that make me nervous (this technique is called systematic desensitization), and since I can't relax and be nervous at the same time, my problem is solved.

"Behavior modification" is a very scary phrase to a lot of people. It reminds us of Orwell's *1984* because it assumes a certain set of "normal" behaviors; then everyone's behavior must be modified to suit the "normal." A behavioral therapist will deny this definition—after all, he or she will say—it is the client who picks the behavior to be modified and the end goal. The behaviorist just engineers the plan when the goals have been defined by the client. In this way the therapist is absolved from letting *his* or *her* own values interfere. This is just fine if you go into therapy knowing exactly what you want. But most people don't. Then the prejudices the therapist has, especially preconceived notions about the adjustment of women to their roles, come into the therapy. If you say to your (behavioral) therapist, "I'm a housewife and have great kids and husband, but for some reason I'm nervous and restless all the time, and I don't know what to do," the response to this is predictable—particularly if the therapist holds the traditional societal views of women. He or she will wind up trying to get you to adjust to the role of housewife. If you have a job and feel you're discriminated against as a woman and you sometimes get very angry about it, the sexist behavioral therapist will probably initiate a program to lower your angry and anxious reaction to discrimination. He or she will teach you to relax to verbal cues like "that dumb bitch" or "women in an office are only good for typing." Then, since the result of this therapy will be the elimination of your "unwanted response," the sexist behavioral therapist will claim to have solved your problem. If you are a lesbian, the heterosexist behavioralist will attempt to make you feel disgusted at the sight of a woman's body so that you will direct no more erotic feelings toward women.

It really comes down to this—the behavior modification therapy you are likely to run into on an out-patient basis is really like any other therapy—as good as the therapist who is using it. If you meet a therapist who seems to be an understanding human being who does not have a preconceived notion of what a woman's life should be, don't run away from him or her just because some behavior modification techniques are used. Chances are he or she will use them only on very specific behaviors *you* want to change and use other forms of therapy to deal with more general problems. But remember, a strict behavioral therapist will not really go deeply into your feelings on any problem. So if these feelings or your struggling with society's constraints on you as a woman are really important to you as part of your therapy— or if you are not sure of the goals of your therapy and don't want to trust them to your therapist, go somewhere else. Even if your therapist sees society as a primary cause of your behavior, he/she is not likely to suggest that you go against conventional norms, because the easiest thing to modify will always be *you*.

A clear exception to this danger in behaviorist therapy is represented by feminist therapists who are training women in "assertiveness training" techniques. These therapists start with the assumption that our culture has socialized most women into timid, submissive, quiet, or overtly "feminine" behavior, especially toward men. Even when their own self-interest is at stake (job, salary, something they want to have or do, etc.), many women are unable to "assert" their right to be treated with respect. Feminist assertiveness training uses behaviorist techniques to break down those old patterns of socialization and build up women's ability to assert themselves in a variety of social contexts. Many different kinds of assertiveness training are available, depending on your community. Therapists can teach it in the context of individual or group therapy. There are many training "courses" that meet once a week for a specified length of time and offer only assertiveness training. There are also several books on how to train yourself to be more assertive. However, not all assertiveness training is feminist. Not all therapists using these techniques have eliminated from their "courses" a subtle double standard of acceptable assertive behavior for men and women. If you decide to try an assertiveness training program, you will still need to evaluate very critically your therapist's assumptions about what is "healthy" behavior for women.

VARIOUS SCHOOLS OF THERAPY

In the last twenty years or so there has been a trend toward the development of new techniques in therapy—for example: primal scream therapy, transactional analysis, client-centered therapy, psychodrama, bioenergetics, sex therapy, goal therapy, group therapy, sensitivity training, sociodrama, role-playing, dance and music therapy, and gestalt therapy. Most of these and other therapies have been designed to explain a specific technique, but unlike traditional models of psychotherapy, they do not place a heavy emphasis on theories explaining personality development. Because of this, such therapies may appear to be nonsexist. But when these therapies are used for women who are confused about sex roles, sexuality, and their identity as women, this absence of theory can itself limit the success of therapy. Women in conflict with society need some analysis of how cultural norms and institutions shape their confusion, and interact with their individual strengths and weaknesses. Without this analysis, a woman can easily fall into the trap of seeing her problems as uniquely her own—if she can't adjust, she is to blame.

Another concern with the new forms of therapy involves the therapists themselves. Whatever techniques your therapist uses, you are still dealing with a person who has been socialized in an extremely sexist society. No one technique or label can by itself assure you that a therapist is open-minded about lifestyles, sympathetic to the position of women in this country, or aware in his or her own life of how deep-seated all our subliminal expectations for men and women are.

FOOTNOTES

[1]Germaine Greer, *The Female Eunuch* (New York: Bantam Books, 1970), p. 92.

[2]Sigmund Freud, "Femininity," in *New Introductory Lectures*, trans. James Strachey (New York: Norton, 1964), p. 113. We added the italics to emphasize Freud's appeal to scientific objectivity.

[3]See Freud's lecture on "Femininity," in *New Introductory Lectures*, pp. 112-35, and his "An Example of Psychoanalytic Work," in *An Outline of Psychoanalysis*, trans. James Strachey (New York: Norton, 1949), pp. 80-99.

[4]Freud, *An Outline of Psychoanalysis*, p. 107.

[5]Freud, *New Introductory Lectures*, p. 128.

[6]Ibid., p. 134. See pp. 132-33 for Freud's discussion of women's lack of contribution to civilization.

[7]Sylvia Plath, *The Bell Jar* (New York: Bantam Books, 1971).

[8]Erik Erikson, "Inner and Outer Space: Reflections on Womanhood," *Daedalus*, 93 (1964), 582-606; as cited in Naomi Weisstein, "Psychology Constructs the Female, or the Fantasy Life of the Male Psychologist," reprinted in *Roles Women Play: Readings Toward Women's Liberation*, Michelle Hoffnung Garskof, ed. (Belmont, Cal.: Brooks/Cole, 1971). Neo-Freudians Karen Horney and Alfred Adler are important exceptions to the perpetuation of Freudian theories about women.

[9]Joseph Rheingold, *The Fear of Being a Woman* (New York: Grune & Stratton, 1964), p. 714; see Weisstein's discussion of Rheingold, ibid., p. 69.

[10]Erich Neumann, *The Origins and History of Consciousness* (Princeton, N.J.: Princeton University Press, 1954), p. 40.

[11]Ibid., p. 175.

[12]M. Esther Harding, *Women's Mysteries* (New York: Bantam Books, 1971), pp. 11, 17.

[13]*The Collected Works of C. G. Jung*, ed. Herbert Read, Michael Fordham, Gerhard Adler, William McGuire; trans. R. F. C. Hull. Bollingen Series XX. Vol. 7, *Two Essays on Analytical Psychology*, copyright © 1953, 1966 by Princeton University Press, pp. 209-10. Short selections reprinted by permission. Originally appeared in *The Relations Between the Ego and the Unconscious*, 1928.

[14]Ibid., p. 209.

[15]Ibid., p. 208.

[16]Ibid., p. 208.

[17]Ibid., p. 209. Jung claims that the models of individuation are exactly parallel and that women should not suppress the animus. But given his description of the animus, his claim is not borne out by his entire theory.

[18]Ibid.

[19]*The Collected Works of C. G. Jung*, ed. Herbert Read, Michael Fordham, Gerhard Adler, William McGuire; trans. R. F. C. Hull. Bollingen Series XX. Vol. 17, *The Development of Personality*, copyright © 1954 by Princeton University Press, p. 198. Short selections reprinted by permission. Originally appeared in *Marriage as a Psychological Relationship*, 1925.

CHAPTER **7**

Choice
and Interaction
in Therapy

The criticisms of therapy that have been presented in this book are not meant to keep you away from therapists altogether. Everyone faces difficulties, and for some, therapy is a means of dealing with them. But we hope we have encouraged you to be more critical in the event you do choose therapy. Understanding the issues that frame the therapy situation will help you as you evaluate your needs, determine your situation, and choose your therapist. However, on a more practical level, you will have some choices and decisions to make about how to find a therapist and how to interact with the therapist you have chosen.

FINDING A THERAPIST

Choosing a therapist should not be a snap decision. Even in the more physiological fields of medicine, people are being advised to interview the doctor before making a definite decision. This interview process is all the more important in the choice of a therapist, because the therapeutic situation in particular is deeply affected by the *assumptions and values* a therapist holds.

One of the best things you can do is to talk with other women who are or have been in therapy and find out their reactions to their specific therapists. But don't stop there. Because a therapist is good for one woman doesn't necessarily mean that that therapist is right for you. During your first visit with a therapist, try to discover just what his or her values and presuppositions about women are. Because of the nature of therapy, it is impossible for a therapist's values— whether professionally or personally based—*not* to play an important role in a woman's therapy. Beware of the therapist who claims to be value-free or objective. Keep in mind what Irene Javors and Charlotte Schwab, Co-Directors of the Feminist Center for Human Growth and Development, have written:

> All therapies are based on value systems. Existing therapies and therapists usually are reluctant to acknowledge this fact. Most therapies claim to be based on scientifically established truth.
>
> Unfortunately, there exists no ONE TRUTH—no undisputed theories and practices. There is extensive disagreement within psychiatry and psychology as to what constitutes "mental health or illness," "normalcy," and "deviancy".... Many therapists ... are using unsubstantiated theories and "truths" to impose their values on *You— The Consumer*! These "bogus scientific systems" are legitimized because those using them have succeeded in getting the state to recognize them as credible [through licensing procedures]. They reflect and reinforce dominant societal values which are sexist, racist, ageist and elitist.[1]

Javors and Schwab go on to suggest that you evaluate potential therapists at least partially in terms of how closely matched your value systems are. We cannot provide a list of specific questions that every woman should ask a therapist she is interviewing because no one set of questions will be applicable to the differing life situations and problems of all women. However, Javors and Schwab have designed a checklist called "Choosing a Therapist: A Non-Sexist Values Checklist." It should provide some concrete direction so that you can, in their words, "identify your own values and a therapist's values so that you may evaluate and decide if a therapist is for you."

In determining your therapist's values, you may want to consider a number of factors that often significantly color the perspective of any therapist—sex, race, class background, religion, age, and sexual orientation. Like anyone else, therapists vary enormously in their ability to transcend their own experience and to empathize with the context and perspective of someone whose background is significantly different.

Sex of Your Therapist

Should you go only to a woman therapist on the assumption that any male therapist who has grown up in this culture will be unable to understand your feelings or help you achieve autonomy? This is an important question for you to answer as you look for a therapist. When you consider that women therapists have been socialized by the same cultural norms that condition their male colleagues, however, you can see that choosing a therapist *solely* on the basis of sex is potentially dangerous. Like men, women have internalized traditional concepts of gender identity and sex roles. These values can color a woman therapist's interaction with you just as they do with male therapists. In fact, some women therapists have imposed traditional norms on their "patients" even more rigorously than male therapists because of their difficulty in gaining acceptance in a male-dominated field.

One woman who went to a woman therapist told us that she felt specially hurt by her therapist's rigidity—it hurt more *because* it came from a woman. She went on to describe her therapist:

> *When I felt I was going off the deep end I went to see a therapist. I was really depressed. She gave me a personality test and a vocational*

CHOOSING A THERAPIST: A NON-SEXIST VALUES CHECKLIST*

Yes	No	My Values	Yes	No	The Therapist
___	___	1. It is important I feel comfortable with my therapist.	___	___	1. My therapist relates to me as an equal human being.
___	___	2. It is important that my therapist be open and honest with me.	___	___	2. My therapist seems open and honest with me.
___	___	3. I feel it is my right to expect my therapist to respect my questions.	___	___	3. My therapist relates to me directly and does not evade my questions.
___	___	4. I need a therapist who will validate my feelings.	___	___	4. My therapist validates my feelings.
___	___	5. I want a therapist who acknowledges that growing is painful and that I am not "sick" or "deviant" because I am in therapy.	___	___	5. My therapist does not label, diagnose or "treat" me as less of a human being because I am in therapy.
___	___	6. I want a therapist who acknowledges and supports me for my decision and self-awareness in seeking therapy.	___	___	6. My therapist is validating and supportive of my decisions and self-awareness.
___	___	7. I want a therapist who encourages me to be self-assertive in the therapy relationship and who helps me to direct the course of my therapy.	___	___	7. My therapist encourages me to be actively involved in my therapy.
___	___	8. I want a therapist who does not reinforce dependency.	___	___	8. My therapist encourages me to be self-dependent.
___	___	9. I want a therapist who does not mystify, but who explains the techniques she suggests.	___	___	9. My therapist teaches me to use techniques so that I can become my own therapist.

CHOOSING A THERAPIST: A NON-SEXIST VALUES CHECKLIST* (Cont.)

Yes	No	My Values	Yes	No	The Therapist
——	——	10. I want a therapist who respects my experience and knowledge.	——	——	10. My therapist respects me as a person with my own unique life-experience.
——	——	11. I want a therapist who does not use her/his degrees to establish competency thereby placing herself/himself on a pedestal distanced from me.	——	——	11. My therapist regards her/his skills as tools with which to help me help myself.
——	——	12. I feel that degrees and credentials do not necessarily make a therapist a helping person.	——	——	12. My therapist does not categorize me within the framework of traditional, sexist training.
——	——	13. I feel that it is important for my therapist to validate me as I am and not try to fit me into a pre-scribed gender role.	——	——	13. My therapist does not view women as having to be passive, sub-missive, dainty, dependent, etc., or men as having to be dominant, aggressive, controlling, self-assured, etc.
——	——	14. I want a therapist who will not try to adjust me to traditional roles as wife, mother, submissive daughter, or as husband, provider, dutiful son.	——	——	14. My therapist views any roles that I may choose as valid and as authentic for me, and helps me to see my choices.

test. She said I was really sick and should be hospitalized. She never cared that I thought I was pregnant. She said I never resolved things with my father. She couldn't help me until I resolved things with my father. She said I would never be able to relate to men until she solved my problem.

Some women, on the other hand, may be so angry about the discrimination they have had to face in their professional life that they will be immediately sympathetic to your problems. Such women may be able to empathize with you much more quickly and more deeply than a man—especially if you want to talk about sex, pregnancy, childbirth, abortion, rape, problems of being a wife or mother, fear of success, and all the other experiences you encounter because you are a woman. Even though a male therapist may be nonsexist, sympathetic, and genuinely sensitive, he is on the other side of the sexual fence. He has had no direct experience that will help him understand many of the things you are talking about.

You can see that it is difficult to decide whether your therapist should be a man or a woman. For example, here's a conversation we had about this subject while we were preparing this book:

Ev: I would go to a woman therapist over a man any day.

Susan: Not me. Depending on their backgrounds, some women are more sexist than men. I would rather go to feminist male therapist than a superprofessional woman on the make or a traditional therapist who happened to be a woman.

Ev: I would trust a woman first. She's a woman—you could always appeal to that in her. You can't do that with a man. You might be able to change a woman therapist; you could disagree with her more easily because she is more likely than a man to understand the problems women have.

Susan: I don't think I agree. I worked for a Black teacher once who hated her Black students' dancing and jiving around. She told me to teach them Shakespeare. The white staff in this program was closer to the students than she was. Some Jews have so many prejudices against Hassidic Jews that they could never deal fairly with them as therapists. I think it's the same with women. I believe a man can change enough by reading, talking to women, and by fighting the traditional values in his own life. I would rather trust a man like this than Hélène Deutsch, as much as I admire her strength.

Ev: If you had only the Yellow Pages to go by, which would you pick? I'd always pick the woman.

Susan: I guess I would, too. I would much rather go to a woman therapist, if I had to choose between a man or a woman I trusted. But I don't think anyone should go by Yellow Pages. Grapevines are better. And I wouldn't trust a woman therapist just because she's a woman. I would want to figure out where she's at just as much as a man.

Ev: I don't think I could ever go to a male therapist.

Susan: If I had problems about sex or childbirth, or abortion especially, I see what you mean. But I still wouldn't go to any woman before any man.

Susan, Cindy, Linda, Nancy: Well, what are we going to say about this in the book?

We never stopped arguing back and forth about whether to recommend only women therapists. In the end, this is something you'll have to decide for yourself. But if some therapist or friend tells you that you should see a male therapist because you are having trouble relating to men, don't accept that theory easily. Both women and men tend to prefer male therapists—because they believe men are more natural authority figures, people with answers—and lots of people think they want this. Instead of accepting this, you should ask yourself what reasons you have for wanting either a man or a woman. Try to figure out whether the sex of your therapist is important to you; try to determine which sex you would feel more comfortable with. When you make a decision, follow through—look for a woman only, if you have decided that is best for you. Or, if you are dealing with a service—such as a clinic—specify right away whether you want a woman therapist or a man therapist. Many psychological services will try to give you what you ask for.

Race of Your Therapist

If you are a minority woman, you cannot afford to evaluate potential therapists only in terms of their sex and sensitivity to women's issues. As minority women in this society, you face the double bind of dual oppression—both racism and sexism have created institutions, attitudes, and stereotypes which limit your potential to become a whole human being. If the therapist you are considering is white, sensitive to white women's problems, but either blatantly racist or simply ignorant of the special history, culture, and needs of various minorities in this country, then you are likely to have to do a lot of explaining before this therapist can really help you with your problems.

White women and minority women share many common issues and experiences—sex roles, child care, work in the labor force, class, rape, beating, birth control, abortion, sexuality, negative images and beliefs about women in the dominant culture, and so forth. But white women's and minority's women experience with these common issues can be very different. Often, the minority woman's problems have been compounded and reshaped by racism; and different conditions have channeled women in different directions. For example, *all* women's experience of their own bodies and sexuality has been deeply injured by the culture's ideal standard of beauty; but minority women have been doubly bombarded because the primary model of beauty has been white.

Because of both race and class differences many Black and white women have grown up with different sex role norms. Many a middle-class white girl subliminally expects that one day some modern "Prince Charming" will come and sweep her of her feet—carry her off into a protected and secure future where she will care for the home while he goes out to work. Depression and the need for therapy often emerge when she begins to realize that this fairy-tale future will never come true. In place of the protecting arm of her husband, she often desires to assert herself as a separate, strong, self-supporting individual. The expectations of many Black girls, however, emerge out of the history of slavery and the continued fact of racism. Particularly for those who grew up in poor families, the fantasy of a protected future is not the predominant fairy-tale of childhood. More often than middle-class white women, Black women have expected to be and have had to be independent and strong in a variety of settings. White therapists who do not understand this different history may perceive this strength as "castrating" and "matriarchal" or may be insensitive to the kinds of problems a Black woman might bring into therapy.

The issue of rape also illustrates the different perspectives of Black and white women that can create misunderstanding in a therapy situation. A Black woman who has been raped by a white man carries with her not only all the current problems of white rape victims, but also a whole historical context of systematic rape and sexual abuse by white men during slavery and up through the present. She may have difficulty expressing her feelings to a white male therapist, particularly if he is ignorant of this history. A white woman therapist may be equally insensitive to another aspect of that history: White women, forbidden as sexual companions to black men, have sometimes falsely accused Black men of rape and contributed to the bloody history of lynching mobs in this country. This racial chasm between Black and white women could easily establish a nontrusting therapy situation.

Minorities other than Black women face similar chasms of experience: Latina, Asian-American, Native-American, Chicano women, and so forth. Therapists who are unaware of cultural and historical differences may inadequately analyze the nature of minority women's problems and the possibility of change. The gap between therapists and minority women may be so great that it inhibits the creation of an atmosphere in which minority women can grow. Therapists who add to their ignorance of minority cultures with damaging stereotypes are likely to be particularly destructive.

If you are a minority woman looking for a therapist, the most obvious solution for you is to find a good minority therapist who is also sensitive to women's issues. But here is where you are caught in the vicious circle of racism. There are few women therapists, but there are even fewer minority people who have made it through the system. If you cannot find someone whose experience and culture is close to yours, then try to find a therapist who is willing to *admit* his or her ignorance and who is *open* to learn as much as possible from you about these differences. You should be able to tell from your first session with a therapist whether he or she sees you as an individual or as a type. Be prepared, however, to be *assertive* about explaining your different experience and needs. Avoid internalizing your therapist's ignorance or prejudice as your own inadequacy.

Class of Your Therapist

Particularly if your socio-economic circumstances are different from your therapist's, his or her class background can deeply affect the capacity to understand the nature of your problem and the options open to you. Whatever your therapist's class origins, his or her profession has most likely created a solid footing in the upper middle-class or upper-class lifestyle. The financial stability and social prestige made possible by high fees may make your therapist stereotype you as a member of a "lower" class or ignore important economic factors in an analysis of your problems.

Class-related issues can create a double jeopardy situation for poor and working class women just as racism does. Sex stereotyping compounded by severe financial stress and low paying, unfulfilling work places a double strain on women for whom the decision to work outside the home is a matter of survival. The therapist who cannot transcend his or her own perspective based on a more secure and prestigious position will have difficulty understanding this double jeopardy and posing possible routes for change.

A few examples will make the problems originating in different class backgrounds more clear. Let's imagine a working-class married woman who has always worked outside the home. Her paycheck is just as important as her husband's for the family's survival, but traditional sex roles in the home have added enormous pressure to her life. She serves double time as worker and wife/mother while her husband enjoys the perquisites of male privilege by relaxing in front of the TV every night. Finally she cracks under the pressure, torn by anger, exhaustion, and fear that she is not being a good wife and mother. She goes to a therapist whose wife is a homemaker, a therapist who accepts traditional sex roles and definitions of masculinity and femininity. He may openly or covertly suggest to her that she is very "threatening" to her husband because her salary is close to his, that her competence at work and home makes him impotent. She should try to be more "feminine," more sensitive to his emotional needs. She should avoid competing with him and instead allow him to be the king in his own house.

His suggestions reinforce the cultural norms that define the ideal (middle-class) family as one where the wife devotes full time to her career of motherhood and wifehood while her husband brings home the paycheck and advances steadily up the ladder of success. Now she feels guilty as an inadequate woman and somehow "inferior" as a member of the working class. This may sound extreme, but we think in reality it is not. A traditional therapist who has a model of mental health in his head that equates femininity with dependence and passivity is likely to see a working class woman's financial independence and assertiveness as "unfeminine." Traditional sex roles (and the established concepts of "mental health" based on them) contain a hidden class bias. The ideal "masculine" breadwinner and "feminine" homemaker contain an assumption of middle-class status that is by definition inapplicable to married women who hold a job out of sheer economic necessity.

Women who are single heads of household may suffer from a therapist's ignorance of class-related issues even more than her married working-class sisters. A woman on welfare, for example, may meet with subtle stereotypes from her therapist, a coded message that she is lazy, careless about her children, promiscuous, unstable, and so forth. Because most therapists are well meaning people who care about their clients, such notions often operate at a subliminal level, but they can color a therapist's concept of a woman on welfare and contribute to a destructive therapy situation. In addition, insensitivity to and ignorance of economic hardship, educational lacks, and social stigma can make it difficult for a therapist to help a woman on welfare to independence, self-confidence, and security. Imagine, for example, that a woman therapist from an upper middle-class background has defied traditional sex roles in her own personal and professional life. With the pressure of career and family greatly relieved by frequent babysitters and cleaning help, she divides the remaining childcare and housework responsibilities somewhat equitably with her husband. Her work is enormously fulfilling. Her salary provides her with a strong sense of economic independence, and she avoids the worst psychology of "mother guilt" because her children attend a superbly staffed and costly day care center. If she is unaware of the options open to her because of her socioeconomic class, she may be unable to offer much help to a woman on welfare. For many women supported by ADC (Aid to Dependent Children), their "options" include menial, not fulfilling, work; continued economic insecurity, not financial independence; the chance to *be* a domestic worker, not *hire* one; destructive child care, not loving, well-funded day care centers; the stigma of being poor and divorced/separated/unmarried, not the support of a husband who is trying to dissolve the prison of sex roles. Such a therapist and such a woman on welfare may be unable to bridge the chasm of class difference to create a good therapy situation.[2]

Not all single heads of household are on welfare of course. There are many women who carry the double burden of being a single parent and holding down some low-paying job with no chance for advancement. For a final example, however, let's take a recently divorced middle-class homemaker who is confronted for the first time with having to support her three children and herself. Child support payments (when made) may provide some money, but not nearly enough. If she has a college degree, she may be lucky enough to find some employment that uses her educational background. But sex discrimination in the work force has established that the main occupation open to women without advanced degrees is clerical. If she has no office skills, she could apply for such jobs as saleslady, bank teller, waitress, grocery clerk, and so forth. Whatever job she finds, her pay will be low and her chances of advancement slim. Without her middle-class husband, her class status will take a plunge even if her class identification remains the same. She will no longer have the money to maintain her former lifestyle, and this tenuous position is likely to produce special tensions that compound the difficulties of being a single, aging woman in American society. A therapist insensitive to these class issues might suggest options based on her former economic status—for example, "You need to treat yourself to some time alone. Hire a babysitter and take a vacation for a couple of weeks"; or "If your children hate their summer babysitter, why don't you send them to camp"; or "If you can't help your kids with their homework at night because of the housework, why don't you hire a cleaning lady."

If you identify with any of the women in these examples, or if you expect that your socio-economic situation is quite different from your therapist's, then your evaluation of your therapist should take into account these class-related issues. You may not be able to find a therapist with a class background like your own. But finding a therapist who has been sensitized to the different needs and experiences of working class people can help prevent destructive therapy. Remember —the full range of difficulties in your *situation* as a working class woman must be understood if therapy can help *you* devise ways of coping with and changing your situation as much as any individual can in an unjust society.

Sexual Orientation of Your Therapist

If you are either a lesbian or uncertain of your sexual orientation, you will want to select your therapist with particular care. In Chapter 4, we outlined a number of cultural stereotypes about lesbians that many therapists, like the general population, still believe: the suspicion that lesbians aren't "real" women, but are instead "masculine" women; the belief that sexual and emotional fulfillment are impossible for lesbians; the fear that lesbians are highly promiscuous and likely to seduce or rape other women, particularly young girls; the notion that lesbians always play male and female roles (butch and femme); the hope that a lesbian experience is just a "stage" that a "feminine" woman will outgrow; and finally the conviction that lesbianism is a form of deviance or mental illness that should be corrected if possible.

The Gay Rights movement, emerging around 1969, and Lesbian Political Feminism (a "branch" of the women's movement) has brought the anger against these stereotypes and an affirmation of gay human rights out of the closet and into the consciousness of many Americans. As a result, there are certainly a number of heterosexual therapists who have sought to eliminate homophobic responses in their own heads so that they can work without fear or prejudice with either gays or the subject of homosexuality itself. But homophobia, the fanatic fear of homosexuality, is widespread in American culture. Especially when colored by fear, stereotypes do not vanish overnight, no matter how well-meaning a therapist might be. And many therapists continue to believe that lesbianism is a form of "mental illness," "sick" behavior that indicates the need for professional "help." Fear campaigns against the basic human and civil rights of homosexuals (like the Anita Bryant "Save the Children" campaign) often justify their position by highly selective use of the Bible to prove that God declared homosexuality to be a "sin." Their attempt to legislate against what they perceive as "sin" imposes their religious beliefs on all others and poses a serious threat to the constitutional separation of church and state. Although therapists who believe their professional theories to be "scientific" would resent the comparison, we believe that the psychiatric designation of homosexuality as "sickness" parallels the religious denunciation. In different language, both reflect the deep-seated homophobia in American culture. While the right-wing campaigners threaten civil rights, prejudiced therapists present a more subtle danger to lesbians and gay men.

A homophobic therapist can reinforce cultural prejudice to make you feel guilty, inadequate and inferior about your erotic feelings for and love relationships with other women. If you are feeling conflicted about your sexual orientation, the therapist's professional "judgment" that you are "sick" can be devastating. If you are quite content about being a lesbian and come to therapy for other concerns, you may discover that the therapist will be unable to meet your needs because of the barrier of prejudice.

The best solution for you is to find a good gay therapist. If you have no idea how to locate a gay therapist, ask lesbians or gay men in your community. Or see if there is a gay rights movement in your area. They will most likely have a list of gay therapists or open-minded heterosexual therapists.

Should you go to a gay male therapist rather than a female nontraditional therapist? Because of common experiences, one might more readily understand your perspective as a lesbian; the other, your situation as a woman. If you are faced with this choice, interview both of them to see with whom you are more comfortable—many gay men have little understanding of the double bind of being both lesbian and female in a sexist *and* heterosexist society; and many heterosexual feminists are *still* uptight about lesbianism.

If there are no gay therapists in your community, then you should interview potential therapists carefully. See what they say about your sexuality. Just as important, see how they relate to you—with nervousness or ease? With subtle stereotyping or openness? In the course of therapy, be prepared to help your therapist out by clarifying the differences in your perspective and experience.

What Is A Good Therapist?

Lesbian women, old women, women of different ethnic and religious heritage, and handicapped women all face the same general difficulties characteristic of minority and working-class women looking for a therapist. But locating a therapist whose values, attitudes, and background are compatible with your own will not ensure that this person will be a good therapist for you. Personal qualities and skills are also important, and *you* are really the only person who can determine the type of person you will be the most comfortable with.

In spite of this inevitable variation, we attempted to determine the common qualities associated with "good" therapists among the many women we talked with. One trait was expressed over and over again: a good therapist is one who lets you discover your own solution, one who doesn't pounce on you immediately with a "diagnosis" and cure. If your therapist claims to know exactly what's wrong with you and exactly how to fix it, go somewhere else. About this type of therapist, Cynthia Cekala wrote:

> The shrink was very nice, white, male, about 65. He asked me about my life, what I believed in, whether I had a sex life, what were the details of it, whether I took drugs, and what I wanted to accomplish. I saw him four times. His advice to me consisted of going to dances at Penn and meeting young law students and staying away from black men. On the fourth time he told me and my mother that I had

schizophrenic reactions due to drugs and two months to two years in a hospital would fix me all up. . . . My admitting diagnosis was "sexual acting out—if not hospitalized might get pregnant or get VD."[3]

Women talked to us about therapists who seemed to have a basic respect and liking for them as people; such therapists listened to what a woman said was the problem instead of telling her what it was, and not respecting her view of the situation. *Warmth, respect, openness, caring,* and *encouraging* are the words that were most often used to describe good therapists, whatever their methods. The gestalt school of therapy was particularly praised by several women—especially because it helped them learn to express anger (punching pillow exercises, psychodrama, and so forth), which is generally a hard thing for many women to do.

Warmth, respect, and caring, however, may not be sufficient by themselves. We have spoken to a number of women who felt frustrated by the "uh-huh" type of therapy. If everything you say is warmly greeted with "That sounds fine," "O.K.," or "good," you may wonder what you're paying all your money for. Acceptance isn't really enough—you also need your therapist's perceptiveness and insight. These are vital if that person is to help you learn to analyze the origins of and potential solutions to your problems. A good therapist most likely has the ability to balance warm, accepting support and nonjudgmental (but sometimes "tough"), perceptive questioning, probing, and pushing to a confrontation with painful feelings.

Because even the best therapy includes arousing raw emotions, it is particularly difficult to evaluate whether your therapist's approach is constructive or destructive. It is easy to describe some ideal balance of warm support and probing analysis in a good therapist, but when *you* face the painful questions you may have trouble deciding whether they can produce growth or regression. Perhaps some perspective on the causes of distress in good therapy situations will help you decide. As we have stated before, we believe a good therapist must understand (and help you understand) the role of societal norms and institutions in the origin of your problems. But you may have responded to your culture with a number of psychological patterns of thought and behavior that are very destructive of your self and/or the people around you. Confronting these patterns and attempting to change can often be painful. Consequently, a notion of the "good" therapist who is *always* 100 percent behind everything you do and say is probably not by itself a good criterion for evaluation. On the other hand, you should avoid a therapist who *continually* justifies all critical comments and questions with an implicit message that he or she "knows what is best for you," knows which questions must be asked and what pain must be confronted. It's the *balance* of respect and insight, warmth and analysis, support and constructive criticism that establishes a good atmosphere for therapy.

A final quality of a good therapist is the recognition that the *situation* of therapy itself is contradictory in nature. Irene Javors and Alexandra Kaplan have described feminist therapy as inherently contradictory, and we would add to their insightful observation that *all* good therapy is similarly contradictory.[4] A good therapist will most likely be aware of these contradictions. Your therapist has extensive training, experience, resources, and a different perspective on your problems—these "qualifications" have brought you to therapy in the first place and they *can* be invaluable. But you and the therapist must avoid the categories "patient" and "doctor," "mentally ill" and "expert," if mutual respect is to develop.

As you seek help in therapy, your sense of your self is probably at a very low, even negative point. But precisely because of this lack of confidence, you are most vulnerable to suffering as a result of bad therapy. Therefore, at your weakest moment, your survival may depend on all the strength and self-esteem that you can muster to determine if a therapist will really help or hinder your growth. As the sessions progress, you rely greatly on your therapist for insight and support while one important goal of therapy is for you to become more independent. Trust must develop between you and your therapist, but your willingness to engage in critical evaluation of your therapist is your best protection against destructive therapy. There is no easy resolution of these contradictions—no magic wand, but only a complex process that will undoubtedly involve conflict and change. But your awareness of these contradictions will help prevent you from becoming trapped by their difficulties. And a good therapist will engage with you in a mutual attempt to transcend these conflicting needs and conditions inherent in the situation of therapy.

Other Problems: Your Location and Your Pocketbook

There are other problems you will have in deciding on a good therapist. For one thing, *where you live* may have something to do with the availability of a variety of therapists. Chances are that you will be more likely to find alternative kinds of therapy in major cities. You will also find a wider range of fees and services in a larger city.

One of the biggest problems you might have in finding a therapist is *money*. Whatever their good intentions or qualities, many therapists are little different from doctors in this regard. Fees of private therapists are often very high—and all too often, fancy homes in the suburbs are built on the unhappiness and need of women and men.

Large fees can be justified and rationalized in all sorts of ways, depending on the therapist. Some undoubtedly think they have worked hard—years of study, training and expense, and so forth—and deserve to make a "decent" living (never expressed as profit) from their "patients." Others say that nothing is as precious as "mental health" or family happiness, so people should be willing to sacrifice to attain these things, just as they would in the case of a physical illness. One feminist therapist at a women's center meeting on women and therapy said that yes, her fees *were* very high—but for professional reasons she had chosen to have her office in a high-rent building so that she could be associated with other therapists. The result was an exceptionally high per-session fee. She also admitted that if she had to choose between two women, she would probably take the one who would pay. Private therapists seldom use sliding scales adjusted to income, and so to pay a large fee you must sacrifice, or be lucky enough to make a large salary, or inherit a lot of money, or have a generous benefactor who is willing to pay (and who might provide the money with strings attached). You can also get health insurance that covers fees for therapists and mental hospitals, but such policies are apt to be expensive.

The result of these typically high fees has been that poor women seldom see private therapists. Phyllis Chesler, in her book *Women and Madness*, says that institutions are filled with poor and third-world women, who for financial or family reasons have been committed without ever having had the option of out-patient therapy.[5] Therapy in this country has been primarily a luxury for middle- and upper-class people.

In some cities there is an alternative to private therapy —some kind of clinic or social service agency. Universities, states, counties, church and social work organizations often have clinics where you can get therapy free, or for a fee determined on a sliding scale. You may be assigned a therapist you can see regularly (not a different therapist every week, as is apt to be the case in medical clinics). Often these therapists work part-time at the clinic and have a private practice or teaching responsibilities as well. Sometimes, clinic therapists are "residents" in training (they will be psychiatrists after three or four years of residency) or graduate students in clinical psychology. The quality of therapists may vary according to the institution, agency, or organization offering the services. And for this reason you must look critically and carefully for a therapist. You will have to devise your own touchstones for evaluation so you can meet your own particular needs, personality, situation, and perspective.

EDUCATING YOUR THERAPIST

No matter how open-minded or easygoing your therapist might seem, he or she has been socialized in the same society you are struggling with. But if your therapist sees you as a person instead of a patient, someone who might have something to teach as well as something to learn, you have a good chance at establishing a constructive, reciprocal relationship.

In spite of the fact that you may feel good about your therapist, remember that he/she is only human—and can be wrong sometimes. Also remember that *you* may be more in touch with your own feelings. Don't be afraid to tell your therapist what's on your mind. For example, let's suppose you are "beautiful" by conventional standards and you are having trouble in your relationships with men because they can't seem to see beyond your looks. Your therapist, whom you feel pretty good about, begins asking you if you are ashamed of your breasts, if you can't talk about sex, if you are frightened or guilty about having intercourse. If you think these questions are off-base, you should say so. See if you can find the strength to tell your therapist "no"—you think the basic problem is the dehumanizing way men look at women and see only bodies; you want your therapist's help in devising ways to force men to see you as a person, to stop yourself from playing the role of the beautiful woman that has probably been reinforced for you ever since you were a pretty baby.

When you disagree with something your therapist says, speak up, but don't just state your doubts and then allow the therapist to take possession of your thoughts and emotions. In particular, when you think he/she is being insensitive to women's problems, say so. Even with the best intentions, your therapist is probably not any more liberated than any of us from the ideas and gut reactions about women we all grow up with. Add to this the layer of training that says therapists are "experts" and people in therapy are "crazy." Be prepared to explain not only *how* you feel, but also *why* you feel the way you do. You may not know why at first. But do your best to discover and back up your reasons. Because you're probably feeling vulnerable, it won't be easy. But it's important to have the courage to "educate" your therapist.

A woman interviewed by Phyllis Chesler explained that this sort of "education" is necessary even for the therapist who thinks of himself or herself as nonsexist. Marilyn told Chesler:

> I'm still seeing a male psychiatrist, and I'm pretty active in the movement.... I think I raised his consciousness the other day.... He [the psychiatrist] was saying that if a therapist really has respect for other people he doesn't need his consciousness raised, he just won't oppress women. I really disagree with that. I gave Dr. X as an example. He used to be a director at a [private psychiatric hospital] and he had a lot of respect for people, sees people as autonomous.... But [even so, he] could say to my supervisor, "I don't know why Marilyn is in women's lib—she's pretty, smart, and feminine."[6]

Therapists have a tendency to say that whatever you're struggling with is *your* unique problem, but you often have to let them know that you're not the only one feeling this way. It might be a good thing to talk about the women's literature you're reading and the women you've confided in.

We realize that this "education" of your therapist may be very hard for you to do, because most women in therapy lack self-confidence and are not feeling particularly strong and forceful. Scorn, dismissal, or patronizing condescension on the part of your therapist in response to your arguments may shrivel you into submission, especially if he or she suggests that your assertiveness is just an intellectualization or a way to escape your "real" problem.

A woman wrote this account of her relationship with her therapist for us:

> *When I went to college, I left behind a family as warm as a cozy nest. Within a year I was deeply in love and soon married. Five years later,*

I was suddenly alone, living in a farmhouse, almost without friends. I beganse eing a therapist because my depression and sense of rejection were so severe. At the same time I was studying existentialism in school. Sartre's portrayal of the hero in Nausea *as fundamentally alone, even in a crowd, really struck me because even as I began making a new life and new friends, I was feeling for the first time in my life that I was* alone, *a separate person, the only person who was going to live my life, however much I might share with other people. It terrified me. A cry in the night. A howl in the wilderness. I couldn't face it, and so I would find myself pacing the farmhouse or putting my head in the corner and staring for hours. I tried to tell the therapist about this and I began by talking about the two kinds of "aloneness" I was experiencing. He became very impatient and said, "All this intellectualizing is just bullshit. You've got to talk about how you feel. Let's get back to your marriage." He was right. It was easier for me to start with Sartre than with the fact that I had stood in the corner for hours feeling like a fat wet worm. But I now wonder if he would have been so scornful to a man who approached his feelings through ideas or literature first. I can't know for sure, but I have heard of some therapists who say that they enjoy a kind of intellectual companionship with their male clients.*

I now wonder what would have happened with a more sensitive therapist, who might have been able to get back to the worm by allowing me to start talking where I could, who wouldn't have shut me up in such a devastatingly scornful way. A therapist tuned in to the problems women have would have immediately recognized this fear of "aloneness," of being a separate person, as crucial to what I was facing in the adjustment from marriage to single life. Now I see so much of the fear and depression I experienced as related to my past underlying belief that a woman alone equals failure and that within a couple relationship, the woman doesn't exist separate from her "wifehood." Certainly my therapist never picked up on any of these issues. If he had understood these things better, he might have been the one to lead me to a new strength. At that time, I certainly didn't have the self-confidence to contradict him. But I like it better as it turned out. Talking to other women with feelings and problems like mine is what is still helping me hammer out a new person, separate but still close to others.

Your therapist's reaction to you when you do disagree may be an important touchstone for evaluating him or her. In any case, the struggle you have with your therapist may end up by making you stronger, more self-confident, and more certain of your identity as a woman. An image of such confidence emerges vividly out of a conversation one woman had with her friend:

JoAnna: You're going to freak out at this, but my therapist keeps telling me that I'm unhappy because I don't dress like a "girl" and I don't fix my hair.
Ruth: How can you stand him saying that?
JoAnna: I just keep telling him he's wrong.

SWITCHING THERAPISTS

At any point during your therapy, you might feel that your therapist is not really helping you. You may feel confused about why you're unsatisfied, and unsure about whose fault this is. You may be wondering if you're just not able to face your problems; or if you're resisting something that might be too painful; or if it's really your therapist who isn't good for you. Your therapist will probably make you feel it's your fault. But don't overlook the possibility that you should look for a new therapist.

There can be some very rational reasons why you're unhappy enough with your therapist to be ready to try somebody else. The problems might be purely individual—a personality conflict. You may feel you can't talk openly with your therapist, that he/she is judging you or reducing you to a psychiatric category of "symptom" or "illness." Or you might feel uncomfortable with some technique he/she is using —behavior modification, touch therapy, transactional analysis, role-playing, etc.

The problem might also be a reflection of the therapist's role in a sexist society. Like you, your therapist has grown up in a culture that designates certain acceptable and narrow roles for women. If you are married, the therapist may expect you to be fulfilled through your husband and children. If you're single, he/she may feel that you are to be pitied because of your supposedly incomplete life. If you work (and more than 40 percent of all women work outside the home), your therapist may see your job as a time-filler, or a way to "help the family out," or as insurance for the future in case your husband dies, or to support yourself because you don't have someone to do it for you.

In addition to therapists' cultural stereotypes of women, their training may have intensified their traditional notions about the development and potential of women. Schools of therapy deriving from Freud, Jung, Erikson, and others have restrictive notions of the role of "normal" women and are part of all psychiatrists' (and most psychologists' and social workers') training. The problems you are having with your therapist may stem from these cultural or professional prejudices.

If you're dissatisfied with your therapy, your first reaction might be to blame yourself. This is a reasonable reaction, considering the role you are being put in—both as a woman and as a person seeking help. But it may not be your fault. Try to think about why the therapy isn't going well, and trust your own judgment. If you think the major problem is with the therapist and not with you, you may decide to quit. At this point most people stop therapy altogether, because the idea of having to start all over again with someone new is too discouraging. But if you still feel you need help—get a new therapist.

Changing therapists may take a lot of courage and self-confidence. Therapists, even those who consider themselves rebels in their profession, tend to side with other therapists. If you are seeing a therapist at a clinic and go above that person's head to an administrator to request a change, the administrator is likely to identify with your therapist and to be suspicious of your reasons ("Are you *really* dealing with your problems?" "Is your therapist upsetting you or are you upsetting yourself?"). When it's a choice between believing you or your therapist, administrators are likely to stop treating you as a human being with problems and start treating you as a "patient" or as a crazy woman, and to believe your therapist. If you are seeing a private therapist and decide to switch to another private therapist, your new therapist may question you very closely about your decision and subtly view your change as a sign of instability. And the more times you try to change therapists, the less believable you become. If your reason for changing is that your therapist is sexist and doesn't understand how your problems relate to social binds, you have even less chance of being believed.

The issue of colleague loyalty is a touchy one with therapists, even those who have been questioning many of the basic premises of their profession. For example, a nontraditional therapist whom we respect and considered nonsexist told us that in the psychology clinic she headed, at least half of the staff therapists (graduate students in clinical psychology) were sexist. In assigning people to therapists, she tried to keep this in mind, but inevitably some women were matched with sexist therapists. Later in the interview, we asked her about policies on changing therapists. She said the clinic administrators frowned on this. A person had to give very good reasons to convince those in charge that she was not just running away from her problems. What if a woman asked to change therapists *twice*, we asked. She just shrugged her shoulders—that person, she said, wouldn't have much credibility. Inwardly, we shrugged our shoulders too—didn't this otherwise fine therapist recognize the contradiction: if 50 percent of the therapists are sexist, then a woman has a pretty good chance of hitting two in a row. Her complaint could easily be legitimate, and not evidence that *she* was at fault.

It takes a lot of self-confidence to decide that your therapist is the one who's wrong, and it takes a lot of determination to change therapists. Here are a few suggestions that might be helpful in changing therapists.

1. Keep believing in yourself.
2. Decide whether or not you should speak to your therapist about your dissatisfaction or decision to change therapists.

Consider whether your therapist seems to be the kind of person who would not be defensive if you said you wanted to change. Some therapists take such a decision as a personal rejection and attempt to justify themselves. You should not feel obligated to explain yourself to such a therapist. But others can be quite open-minded and unthreatened by your decision and may be willing to help you locate someone more suitable.

3. Try to decide as soon as possible that you want a new therapist—if you can, make up your mind within a few weeks of beginning therapy. Your credibility is apt to be greater if you and the therapist haven't gone very deeply into your problems yet. Also, it's a real hassle to start explaining your problems from the beginning all over again.

4. If your therapist is associated with a clinic or mental health organization try to find a new therapist at a different place. If you stay within the same institution, your new therapist may identify with your old therapist's point of view, so you won't really be getting a fresh start. Collaboration between therapists and resistance to your desires for change will probably be stronger in small organizations. Even when you do go to a different place for therapy, your new therapist may call your old one to discuss your problems.

5. If you are seeing a private therapist, avoid changing to a therapist affiliated with your old therapist. Many private therapists understandably join together in loose affiliations to share space, facilities and rent and also to have colleagues with whom they can exchange ideas and experiences. But this important sense of community among private therapists can potentially create preconceived notions about you if your old therapist talks about you or shares your file with your new therapist. If your therapist is not affiliated with anyone, simply look for a new therapist who doesn't know your old therapist well (if at all).

6. If you are involved in a service clinic, and *must* stay there, have the change made through the administrators, if possible. Some places require you to confront your therapist before you can see someone else. This may be very hard for you to do, and the therapist may make it even harder. He or

she may tell you that you're not being honest with yourself, or are distorting or running away. This is especially true if you tell your therapist you don't like his or her attitude toward women. But if you really feel you have been honest and accurate in your evaluation, say so. The point is, if you *can* get your therapist changed through administrative channels, it will be easier for you.

A woman told us this about the problems she had in changing therapists at a clinic:

After months with a therapist who was first assigned to me when I was in an in-patient ward of a psychiatry clinic, I finally decided that he was cutting me down instead of giving me confidence. He was making me feel crazy by doubting everything I said. I told him that I wanted to change therapists, and he replied that I would have to go through the intake procedure again. That I did happily and was assigned to a therapist I liked in our first talk. Before my first appointment, he called me up to cancel it, saying that he had talked to my original therapist—who told him that I had tried to seduce him and wanted to leave so I could try it with someone else! I protested, but the new therapist insisted that I work out my problems with my old therapist. I was very upset and confused by his charge, because during therapy he had told me that he had fallen in love with me. When I rejected him, he told me that my basic problem was that I didn't know how to give or receive love.

I didn't try another therapist at the clinic. Instead, I called a private therapist who had filled in once for my vacationing therapist. The appointment was made, but halfway through the week, it was broken by the therapist. I said to her, "So they've gotten to you, too." She answered that she had been talking to my therapist and decided he was right—I should work out my problems with my first therapist. Greatly frightened and needing help, I became hysterical on the phone. The woman relented and gave me the name of a new therapist in town—one none of the others knew.

WOMEN'S GROUPS AND YOUR THERAPIST

If you are a member of a women's group, especially the small, often closed kind of group known as a "consciousness-

raising" or "CR" group, don't be too surprised if your therapist doesn't like the idea. Therapists are likely to see women's
groups as a threat. If you are talking about your problems
regularly with other women in a tight-knit group, the group
will probably be seen as competition by your therapist—just
as your seeing another therapist would be competition.

A graduate student in training to be a therapist told us:

> *When I was in therapy, my therapist, whom I liked and trusted, asked
> me not to join a women's group. We both felt that part of my problems
> involved a desire to dump all my difficulties in my friends' laps. He
> thought being in a women's group would just reinforce my inability
> to deal with problems alone. He felt that he could help me be indepen-
> dent better than a women's group. I was confused and upset; I finally
> decided to do what he said.*

Is this a fair attitude on the part of therapists? If your
therapist is against your being in women's groups, you will
have to decide for yourself. But there are some important
issues at stake that you should understand as you make your
decision.

In the first place, your therapist is right to see women's
groups as competition in some sense. Consciousness-raising
groups—whose purpose is to help women deal with their
problems as women—and also project groups—such as health
collectives—do challenge the traditional way of dealing with
unhappiness through therapy. For some women, such groups
can be a real alternative to therapy. Instead of developing a
dependence on one person (usually male) who has special
training, women within a group—many of whom are facing
the same pressures—help solve each other's problems. Rather
than professional degrees, it is personal experience that quali-
fies them to help. It's no wonder that many therapists see
women's groups as a threat to their professional status. And
for a male therapist, there might be the added threat to his
"masculinity"—that a woman might prefer the help of other
women to him. And, too, some therapists might—consciously
or unconsciously—assume that women have more trouble
than men seeing their problems "objectively." Nineteenth-

century philosopher (and misogynist) Otto Weininger stated blatantly what many people today still believe:

> The feeling of identity . . . is quite wanting in the true woman because her memory, even if exceptionally good, is devoid of continuity . . . women, if they look back on their earlier lives, never understand themselves.[7]

Also, women's groups are acutely aware of the social origins of a woman's difficulties; as a woman tries to talk through her problems, and as the other women in the group question and probe her situation and feelings, an analysis of those problems emerges. And this analysis is likely to be far different from the "diagnosis" of many therapists. Where the therapist might center on personal inadequacy or early childhood, the women's group tends to point to the external pressures, the stereotypes of "feminine" behavior, and the woman's own attitudes toward being a woman. This different focus represents a real threat to traditional therapy, which concentrates on adjusting a woman to societal expectations and norms.

The following story illustrates this sharp contrast between the traditional therapeutic analysis of a woman's problem and the kind of interpretation provided by a women's group. Two freshman roommates became close friends and for a time did everything together. Then one of them fell in love, began to spend all her time with her boyfriend, and finally saw her old friend only to say goodnight. The friend was disturbed by this change in their relationship. So she went to the college psychiatrist. After five minutes, the psychiatrist told the girl that her problem was a bad relationship with her mother and lesbian desires for her roommate. The result: she gained nothing but guilt. This incident occurred years before women began to share their experiences in consciousness-raising groups. But if this woman could have gone to a contemporary woman's group, they would have insisted that she not blame herself for her roommate's "desertion" of the friendship. They would have supported her resentment of the low priority her roommate had placed on her relationship with women friends. They would have pointed out that most women are socialized to believe that their sexual/love relationships with men are more important than their friendships with women. Underlying this coded message is the reality that a woman's legitimate role in society depends upon her ability to get married and stay married. In the unwritten codes of the marriage "marketplace," women learn to compete with other women for male attention and approval. Consequently the bonds of female friendship have often been weak. Seen in this cultural context of dominant values, the roommate had abandoned her woman friend as soon as a man beckoned. The psychiatrist's instant diagnosis reflected societal norms and drove deeper the wedge of self-doubt and guilt in the woman whose friendship had been so abruptly rejected. After helping her to see her experience in the light of a feminist analysis of her situation in its personal and political dimensions, the woman's group would then go on to suggest ways for her to confront her friend or to find friends who treated their relationships with women with respect.

With their explicit feminist analysis of women's lives and the development of a nonprofessional women's support network, women's groups certainly represent a radical alternative to traditional therapy. But therapists' negative attitudes toward women seeking two different kinds of aid at the same time are probably more often based on prejudice and misconceptions about women's groups rather than on a real understanding of the issues at stake. Your therapist may, for example, assume that women's groups are filled with manhating, unhappy women who wouldn't be there if they had "normal" relationships with men. He or she may believe that you are too "political" as a way of "escaping" your personal problems—that is, you blame society for your own failures and join the women's movement to rationalize your "projection." One woman in a psychiatry clinic said that her therapist's reaction to her membership in a woman's group was this comment: "Your woman's group is just part of your craziness!"

Both male and female therapists can be simultaneously ignorant of and defensive about the feminist movement. But if your therapist is a man, the likelihood of his feeling threatened by your association with feminism is probably greater. A therapist discussing women's groups versus therapy drew the hypothetical case of a woman who was having problems getting along with men. He said that a women's group "with all its slogans and cliches" would just reinforce this woman's distrust of men. It would give her an out—she wouldn't have to face her personal failure because everyone in the group would automatically blame men. What the therapist assumed was that all CR groups do little more than foster a simplistic view of men and offer blindly loyal support to women. But in reality, women's groups, on the whole, tend to focus more directly on *women*, rather than on men: the socialization of women; norms for "femininity"; acceptable female roles; institutional forms of discrimination; women's response to an oppressive society (guilt, inferiority complex, male identification, anger, rebellion, etc.). Rather than hunting for scapegoats, most CR groups engage in a process that reverses traditional female socialization and devises ways for women to combat sexism.[8]

Some women told us that therapy is either entirely destructive or so often destructive for women we should advise women to steer clear of all therapy and become involved in a woman's group instead. For example, one woman told us after she finished reading an early draft of this book: "I have had ten years of experience with therapists and mental institutions. I strongly feel that therapy is destructive. I would certainly never go to a therapist again. I hope you will not recommend that women go see therapists. I think a good woman's group can help them much better."

We don't believe, however, that good therapy and women's groups (or any involvement in feminism) are mutually exclusive. Some women may get a certain kind of constructive help from other women and at the same time a more concentrated, directly personal kind of help from therapy. One feminist who was in both a woman's group and private therapy told us that her woman's group has helped her to see her personal problems in the social context of sexism and has given her an ongoing support group of women friends. Therapy, on the other hand, allows her to focus on extended exploration of why she has so much trouble changing old patterns of thought and behavior based on traditional notions of women's roles. To explore herself week after week in her women's group in all the detail that therapy allows would disturb the balance of the group by allowing her needs to take precedence over other discussions. Should you join a women's group at the same time you are in therapy? Should you opt for one alternative over the other? We can't make a blanket recommendation. There is no single answer. A lot depends on the women's group, the therapist, and your assessment of their value to you. And much depends on your own ability to determine just what your needs are.

If you plan to join or continue in women's groups at the same time you go to a therapist, it might be a good idea to ask your therapist what he or she thinks of women's groups. The answer might be a good touchstone for evaluating your therapist.

THE POTENTIAL OF THERAPY: CAN YOU GET HELP ANYWHERE?

Some people who have read parts of our book in manuscript form felt that we have painted an unnecessarily dark picture of what therapy is like today. It is not traditional or male therapists who have made such complaints; for the most part, they have been made by women whose friends and commitments are heavily centered in a daily struggle for change. Some have been feminist therapists or feminists in training to do therapy. These people believe that the situation is not static—that times *are* changing, and it is now becoming possible to find therapists who are challenging the conventional norms for women.

It is true. Times are changing. Attitudes are changing. Women—and not just women who openly identify themselves with the woman's movement—are speaking up. For example, a college teacher said:

> *My literature class, which consists mainly of open admissions students in New York, is not listed as a women's studies course (that would be politically impossible), but as we read literature dealing with rape, marriage, prostitution, double standards, etc., woman's issues inevitably become the explosive center of discussion. All it takes is one or two outrageous comments and the women (and some men too) take up arms and articulately, angrily, gloriously refuse to let such ideas rest undefeated. In my classes in 1968, the women were silent, with few exceptions. I cannot imagine them having spoken with the kind of anger and assurance that many women students today do.*

No matter how much it has been scorned or mocked, the women's movement has had an enormous impact on people's attitudes and expectations for women. A prime-time TV special on women's history in America would never have appeared in 1968, especially as the kickoff for a thirteen-part series of American life. A girl on *Sesame Street* now tells a spider to bug off, saying that "little girls aren't afraid of spiders any more." Many women *and* men are reexamining their views of women in the world. The impact of the woman's movement on a woman's right to control her body has been enormous. Although the controversies stirred by the issues of abortion, sterilization, and birth control are far from settled, more women today are able to assert their right to determine what will happen to their bodies than they were ten years ago. Parent committees and educational agencies are beginning to attack sexism in the schools and to design or advocate nonsexist curricula. Affirmative action guidelines, some federal legislation, government agencies, and equal rights amendments at the state level have begun to establish the legitimacy of equality for women, although the achievement of equality is clearly a long way off and the resistance to change is often enormous.

Yes, things are changing, and the changes are beginning to influence the therapeutic process, however slowly. There is no doubt that even therapists who have been practicing for a long time have begun to feel the impact of these changes, as have the younger therapists who are growing into the profession in the midst of this change. A feminist therapist told us after reading part of our manuscript:

> *I think you don't emphasize enough how much things are changing. Today it's possible to find nontraditional therapists who have radically reversed in themselves the conventional ideas of what men and women should be and do. Women can find help. I myself had a very good experience in therapy. When I first went to my therapist, I sat there and waited for her to tell me what it was I needed and wanted. But right from the first, she refused to give me answers or let me develop that kind of dependence on her. She insisted that I must find out for myself what I wanted to experience, what kind of a person I wanted to become. On this very fundamental issue, she forced me to develop the strength to make my own decisions about the direction of my life. She gave me power. Or rather, she taught me how I could become a powerful person. Independent. Potent. Before therapy, I was unable to make even the smallest decisions. Now I decide. I can feel and live my own power.*

A feminist in training to be a therapist reinforced this confidence in nontraditional therapy by saying:

> *I think it's important that you give women a feeling that they can find help somewhere. I've certainly gotten a lot of help from my therapist. I started seeing a male therapist with my husband a year and a half ago. We had been married almost ten years and had two young children. I was just beginning to go back to school again, just getting away from being a compulsive housekeeper and mother, but our lives had grown apart. My husband and I started to see this gestalt therapist to try to work through our marriage difficulties. For a long time,*

I felt that the therapist was really committed to the marriage—that he was working to get us adjusted to each other, whatever the cost. I I couldn't believe for a long time that he really saw me as a person separate from my marriage. But after I began to see this therapist myself, I gradually came to feel that he really did care about my individual development. As I began exploring my feelings of wanting to live separate from my husband—not only by having a job and splitting child care but also by having separate rooms and finally separate homes—and to try a sexual relationship with a woman, I found that my therapist did not judge my lifestyle by his own. He really seemed completely at ease with my trying anything I wanted. He did not impose his ideas on me. Instead, I have been able to talk through with him all my feelings, many of them mixed and uncertain as well as positive and exhilarating. He has been a great support in this way. As my separation becomes a reality, I will need him to talk about my feelings during the difficult adjustments for myself and my children.

At the forefront of this move to make therapy sensitive to women's issues and beneficial to women's search for strength in a hostile society have been psychologists who advocate major change in the mental health system. Psychologists associated with the school called Radical Therapy have been publishing for some years a journal (named *The Radical Therapist*, then *Rough Times*, and currently *State and Mind*) and various books attacking therapy as an institution that promotes adjustment rather than change. Women in the field of psychology have adopted a number of strategies to raise awareness of gender issues: publish the *Psychology of Women Quarterly*; work within the various professional organizations of psychologists and psychiatrists to change the concepts of mental health and the kind of therapy women are likely to get; and form their own division within the American Psychological Association. A new school of therapy has emerged from a decade of scholarship and political organization: Feminist Therapy. It takes the perspectives of feminism and applies them to the therapeutic situation—that is, to both the content and process of therapy. Elizabeth Friar Williams has defined a feminist therapist as:

one who helps a woman examine how she learned from the culture the behaviors and emotions expected of her as a "normal" woman: behaviors and emotions she now may find bar achievement of her full potential as a competent person and fulfilled lover.[9]

Feminist scholars Diane Kravetz and Jeanne Marecek have described the goals of feminist therapy as "helping women to discover their personal strengths, to achieve a sense of independence, to view themselves as equals in interpersonal relationships, and to respect and trust themselves and other women." They go on to summarize the field of feminist therapy:

> The development of feminist therapy reflects the conviction that personal change and sociopolitical change are inextricably linked. Thus, in feminist therapy, identifying sexism and its effects on the client and other women is an important and active ingredient of the treatment process. The relationship between the goals of treatment and social change is emphasized through discussion of the ways in which the social roles and rights of women influence the client's personal experiences. Significant social change is understood as a necessary substrate for many areas of individual change.

> Another hallmark of feminist therapy is its commitment to feminist principles, including self-help, collective rather than hierarchical structures, and equal sharing of resources, power, and responsibility. Therapeutic strategies are chosen to be consistent with these principles, because it is assumed that helping women to change the oppressive aspects of their lives outside the therapy situation requires eliminating the oppressive aspects of therapy as well. For example, modes of therapy that place clients in subordinate roles to an authoritarian therapist echo women's inferior status in society. Therefore, feminist therapists deliberately select therapeutic strategies that emphasize client's power and responsibility.[10]

As a result of the efforts of feminist therapists and others committed to change in the profession, it is indeed easier for women to find good therapists. As you search for a nonsexist therapist, however, try to avoid the common stereotypes and misconceptions often associated with the words "radical" and "feminist." Victimized by media distortions, you may eliminate from your list of possible therapists just those ones who will be most open to understanding and helping you with your problems. One feminist therapist told us:

> *Demystify the word "feminist" for your readers. Some women are afraid that a feminist therapist will be hard, strident, and dogmatic and want her clients to become that way. All the false stereotypes of "feminists" in general have been just as falsely applied to feminist therapists. A feminist therapist is not an ogre who hates men and forces women to abandon marriage. The label is much more likely to mean that she will be open to explore with women their urge to develop an identity that does not sacrifice its autonomy to the wishes and demands of men and children.*

Whether or not a therapist identifies herself or himself as a "feminist therapist," there are an increasing number of therapists available today who espouse nonsexist values in therapy. Your community may have a number of resources that can help you locate such therapists. Women's centers and local women's groups often develop lists of good therapists in a given area. A number of feminist referral centers maintain lists of nonsexist therapists. And some areas have organizations rooted in the women's movement that do lay and professional counseling, as well as referrals. Grapevines of women who have been in therapy may also help you to locate a good therapist. If you are willing to spend the time looking carefully, you may be able to find a therapist who has abandoned stereotypes of women, who fights the natural tendency of the therapist to impose explanations and "solutions," whose ideas have not been influenced by traditional psychological training, who has tried to resocialize his or her own attitudes about women—who, in short, is aware of and tries to avoid most of the problems we have warned you of.

But what are your chances of finding a therapist like this? How much have things *really* changed—in *all* parts of the country, for all classes of women? Certainly the change in attitudes has only barely begun to show itself in tangible changes in the economic system, the business world, in the areas involving job opportunities, division of household chores, treatment of lesbians, child care, and so forth. Even if you do find a therapist who can help you to free yourself, you will have to confront the same destructive pressures and situations in a world that has not changed as much as you have. Can an individual be free in an unfree society? Stronger, maybe, but not free.

And has the change in attitudes brought about a really deep, lasting change in the subliminal socialization we have all experienced?[11] How much of this change is merely lip-service—a defensive covering over of deep-seated restrictive assumptions about women that have taken a person's whole life to develop and that certainly cannot be easily reversed by rational decision or even by a few years of conscious effort? For decades, many therapists have insisted that they are "scientists," that they don't approach their "patients" with any assumptions about what they should be. Behaviorists openly declare their objectivity; Freud himself introduced his article on "Femininity" by saying his theories were based on "nothing but observed fact." Given this traditional assertion of objectivity in a strikingly subjective profession, it would be quite natural for many therapists to *say* that they impose no attitudes about women on their "patients"—when in *fact* they do.

A therapist's belief in his or her own objectivity may do little more than force sexist attitudes "underground" where the harm they can do is even greater since both the therapist and the person in therapy believe in the therapist's "neutrality." The danger of so-called "value-free" therapy is evident in the account of a woman who works on Title IX implementation in school districts. She designs guidelines and curricula to help the schools institute equality in education. She reported a conversation with a high school counselor on the influence of his values in the counseling situation. Believing himself able to separate his professional behavior (objective) from his personal value system (subjective), he told her: "I will change my behavior from 9:00–4:00 to comply with Title

IX. But there's no way that my wife will be equal with me at home!" Frustrated, the woman told us: "There's no way he can promote women's equality in his work!" Similarly, therapists who believe in their own "objectivity" and yet do nothing to eliminate their own sexist notions in their private lives have little chance of helping women in therapy.

But many therapists have recognized the impossibility of divorcing their own values from the therapy situation. Many have assumed a nontraditional label or stance in regard to women's roles. But given the difficulty of resocialization to nonsexist values, it is also difficult to believe that labels and position statements can always be taken at face value. To put into practice what one believes intellectually is hard for everyone; and therapists are no exception. How then can women assess a therapist? Even if a therapist claims a nontraditional, feminist-oriented approach, how can a woman find out to what extent this is true? This is a difficult question. In interviewing therapists, we found it next to impossible to devise questions about women that could not be sidestepped by a therapist who might want to give the impression that he/she is sympathetic to the issues raised by the women's movement.

The Feminist Therapist Roster, a national listing of good therapists for women, is an important first step in developing necessary referral systems for women. But the difficulty in building accurate lists is evident in the sparse form sent out to potential therapists for inclusion on the national listing:

Name

Address(es)

Phone

Credentials: (Briefly—degrees, training, licenses, experience, etc.)

Services Offered: (Types of therapy, age groups, specialty areas)

Statement of position on feminism (sentence or two)

Another problem with relying completely on labels is that a therapist may have all the properly open attitudes and *still* be a lousy therapist—or at any rate not the person you can work with. Many of the women we talked to who had had good experiences with therapy simply felt that their therapists were good human beings—they cared, they were warm, they didn't impose diagnoses, they had respect for the troubled persons who came to see them week after week. We do suggest that you hunt out therapists who openly associate themselves with nontraditional and/or feminist therapy, but do not assume that such a therapist will automatically hold all the solutions to your problems. You will still need to keep your eyes open.

Labels are not the only problem in determining how deep the changes have been in the culture. The impact of the woman's movement has been very uneven. The lives of many people, therapists included, in some places have indeed been changed permanently. But you may live in a part of the country where the word "feminist" means something close to "female devil" or "castrating bitch," or where the one feminist therapist in town is set up in private practice without sliding fees, while the public clinic you may have to attend doesn't even have a woman therapist, much less a radical one. Radicals in all professions have trouble getting and holding jobs. For example, how easy is it for a nontraditional therapist to be hired by a large institution controlled by conservative psychiatrists or by a small church-affiliated agency?

Then there is *you*—you may be one of those who feels hostile to anyone connected with the woman's movement. You may, in short, be like the thousands of women who just go to a therapist—any therapist, or your friend's therapist. What will *you* find in therapy? Will it be positive or negative?

If you are afraid you are going to kill yourself, if you are totally isolated, "spaced-out," "freaked-out," out of control, if you feel the urge to "act out" in strange and unacceptable ways, you probably feel you *have* to seek therapy, no matter how slim the chances of finding a nondestructive therapist—

because where else in this society can you get help? Whatever is available, you will take it. What kind of therapy will *you* find?

Answers to these questions undoubtedly vary from community to community, but it is unrealistic to believe that, despite the great changes that have taken place, a woman can easily find a nontraditional or feminist therapist. Whatever therapist you decide to work with, you need to carefully evaluate that person's actions and words. You need to watch out for hidden or blatant limiting assumptions about women. This is no easy task—because at the same time you are experiencing self-hate, lack of confidence, and perhaps even a real urge to run away from your problems, you must be ready to examine and evaluate the validity of your therapist's comments and actions, especially when they run counter to your own feelings. You must have the strength to determine whether or not your therapist is destructive—and if he/she *is*, you must find the strength to quit.

So—you know that finding a good therapist is hard. And evaluating that person once you are *in* therapy is harder. But remember that you have a choice. Don't accept just anyone. Look carefully for the person you can work with, the one who will open doors for you instead of closing you into constricting "feminine" categories that will leave you discontented, guilt-ridden, unhappy, and perhaps worse off than before.

FOOTNOTES

[1] Irene R. Javors and Charlotte Schwab, "No One Has the Right to Classify Anyone," *Majority Report*, 6, no. 25 (16–29 April 1977), p. 5. For further information on the following Checklist and the Center, write: Irene Javors and Charlotte Schwab, Directors, The Feminist Center for Human Growth and Development, Suite 1-C, 40 E. 68th St., N.Y., N.Y. 10021.

[2] See Bev Fisher, "Race and Class: Beyond Personal Politics," *Quest*, 3, no. 4 (Spring 1977), 2–14 for an excellent discussion of the differing needs of middle-class and working-class and/or minority women.

[3] Cynthia Cekala, "If This Be Insanity . . .," *Rough Times*, 3, no. 1 (September 1972), 2. *Rough Times* was first called *The Radical Therapist* and is now called *State and Mind*.

[4] Javors and Kaplan presented their excellent analysis based on discussions in the Androgyny and Mental Health Workshop at the Working Conference on

Androgyny and Sex Role Transcendence in Ann Arbor, Michigan (May 1978). Their work will be published as a chapter in the forthcoming book based on the conference.

[5]Phyllis Chesler, *Women and Madness* (New York: Doubleday, 1972), pp. 306-33. See also Thomas S. Szasz, *Ideology and Insanity: Essays on the Psychiatric Dehumanization of Man* (New York: Anchor, 1970), pp. 82-83, 86; Saul V. Levine, Louisa E. Kamin, Eleanor Lee Levine, "Sexism and Psychiatry," *Psychiatry*, 44, no. 3 (April 1974), 333.

[6]Chesler, *Women and Madness*, p. 259. Excerpts from *Women and Madness* by Phyllis Chesler. Copyright © 1972 by Phyllis Chesler. Reprinted by permission of Doubleday & Company, Inc. and Penguin Books Ltd.

[7]Otto Weininger, *Sex and Character* (1903; rpt. New York: AMS Press, 1975), p. 146.

[8]CR groups vary enormously, of course. For a good general description of one type, see Pamela Allen, "Free Space," in Anne Koedt, Ellen Levine, and Anita Rapone, eds., *Radical Feminism* (New York: Quadrangle, 1973), pp. 271-79.

[9]Elizabeth Friar Williams, *Notes of a Feminist Therapist* (New York: Praeger, 1975), p. 5. See also Anica Vessel Mander and Anne Kent Rush, *Feminism as Therapy* (New York: Random House, 1974).

[10]Jeanne Marecek and Diane Kravetz, "Women and Mental Health: A Review of Feminist Change Efforts," *Psychiatry*, 40, no. 3 (November 1977), 326-27. Their references are an excellent guide to research on women's mental health issues.

[11]For a discussion of subliminal ideologies, see the excellent article, "Training the Woman to Know Her Place: The Power of a Non-Conscious Ideology," by Sandra L. Bem and Daryl L. Bem, in *Roles Women Play: Readings Toward Women's Liberation*, Michelle Hoffnung Garskof, ed. (Belmont, Cal.: Brooks/Cole, 1971), pp. 84-96.

Policies and Procedures in Psychological Service Institutions

As we have discussed in earlier chapters, you may well find that the cost of private, individual therapy is prohibitive. In this case, you will probably find that you have to look for a therapist within some kind of psychological service institution. For this reason this chapter deals with the policies and procedures within typical service institutions. This may help you in your search for the best therapist for your needs.

You should not walk into a therapy situation "blind." You are more likely to have a bad experience with therapy if you are ignorant of such things as how a service is run, the decisions you might have to make before your therapy begins, the often dehumanizing intake procedures, how your file is kept, and so forth. If you're very upset and disoriented when you start looking for a therapist, you can feel terribly helpless in the face of an efficient receptionist or an "intake" therapist who determines after a short talk what kind of therapy you need. If you are armed with certain types of information about the psychological service you are considering, you will feel less helpless and will be less a victim of bureaucratic rules or of an autocratic therapist.

The procedures a particular service uses to get you set up in some form of therapy can tell you many things about the regard that service has for the people who use it. If you know these procedures, you'll have a better basis from which to accept or reject that service. You can gather this type of concrete information without putting your feelings on the line and use it to "shop" at different services. You won't have to wait until you've spent two hours in a waiting room to find out you can't afford a particular service, or that you have to be a student to go there.

Also, from the second you walk in you will be asked to make many decisions that will affect the course of your therapy. You may be asked to decide whether you want group or individual therapy, whether you want a man or woman therapist, whether you will be willing to take drugs or psychological tests, or have your sessions tape-recorded. If you know beforehand what decisions you'll have to make, there will be far less chance that you will be pressured into a bad situation. You'll also become more aware of what decisions are being made for you. Some places, for example, don't ask if you want to take drugs—they offer you the choice between drugs and no help at all.

In trying to gather this type of concrete information in our own community (Madison, Wisconsin), we interviewed personnel (administrators and/or therapists) at approximately twenty services. We tried to get a cross-section of services, both in size and in politics. Before our study began, we decided on a list of topics we felt were most important for a potential "client" to know about. These areas are listed here; they include some generalizations we made from our examinations. We hope you'll find these topic areas and our comments about them helpful in your search for a therapist.

Finding Help

Your first step consists of getting information like addresses and phone numbers. Most places require a potential client to make an appointment, after which it is necessary to wait anywhere from one hour to three weeks to see someone. But it might also be helpful to find out numbers you can call if you need desperately to contact someone for help during non-business hours.

"Intake procedures," as they are so warmly called, vary from assigning you to whoever happens to be around to setting up an intricate series of meetings and interviews. We found only one place in Madison, Women's Place (a nontraditional, lay-counseling service), that allows the "client" to talk to several people, and then lets that person choose someone she feels she can relate to.

If you want to change therapists after therapy has started, most places we investigated will let you do it once—but will give you a hard time. If you try to change again, the attitude is that you are trying to escape reality. Forget trying to change therapists in a small service. The difference in therapists who have to report to the same boss, who see each other constantly, and who may discuss their "clients" with each other will be minimal.

Cost, Eligibility, and Length of Treatment

The importance of cost and eligibility are obvious. Most services we investigated had sliding scales that varied widely according to need. Most services accepted anyone for therapy, although some specified categories such as students only. Services with religious affiliations are usually open to anyone —you don't have to be Catholic to go to Catholic Social Services.

Length of treatment is also important. Are you looking for someone to talk to once or do you need a long-term relationship with a therapist? Most places we studied had treat-

162

ments of varying lengths, from rap centers, which are usually one-shot deals, to long-term arrangements with psychiatrists. Most services specified that they preferred a termination date of at most, six months.

Therapists and Staff

Who is on the staff? How many women? Are they psychologists, psychoanalysts, psychiatrists, psychiatric nurses, vocational counselors, social workers? Each of these labels involves different training and certain biases you should be aware of. At some services, you are likely to get a therapist who is only in training (this may affect the quality of your therapy for better or worse). If you want a woman therapist, you should find out if one is likely to be available at this service; you don't want to go through an exhausting intake procedure only to find out that the one woman therapist is booked up for two years.

Also, try to find out what kind of people go to any particular service. We found that many services either didn't know much about the people they served or were hesitant to give out that information. You should know something about the majority of the people who seek help there. If a lot of women who share some of your cultural and political backgrounds go there, chances are you won't be treated like an alien.

Kinds of Therapy

Ask around to find out what kinds of therapy are available. Does a particular service have a specialized emphasis? Does it, for example, specialize in family counseling? Marital counseling? Group therapy? Or does it offer just about anything? In our study most places offered group *and* individual therapy, but they had little or no experience in therapy for gay couples or groups of people who live or work together. In Madison, almost every service claimed to be "eclectic." Usually, services are reluctant to admit an affinity with any one school (Freudian, gestalt, behaviorist, transactional analysis, Rogerian, Jungian, etc.); and frequently, alternative types of therapy are simply not available in smaller cities. In big cities, it is easy to find services or therapists who openly affiliate with a particular school. If you do find yourself with a therapist who represents a particular school, try to find out something on your own about that school.

Files and Confidentiality

The politics behind this subject are dealt with in Chapter 3. However, you need to be aware that most services *state* a policy—but it is unclear how often the stated policy represents actual practice. This is reflected in the sentence you will see in the descriptions of two of the agencies we describe later in this chapter. It says, *"This service's stated policy is given below—actual practice is unknown."* Keep that in mind.

Tapes, Tests, and Drugs

Most institutions, and especially those that train therapists or are funded by foundations or the government, tape-record their therapy sessions. The agencies we talked to all assured us that they erase these tapes immediately after using them for a specific purpose, such as supervising trainees. However, their actual practice is unknown. They varied in whether or not they allowed a "client" to refuse to be taped—one therapist looked shocked when we suggested that some people might feel too intimidated by the recorder to be honest. In any case, if you don't want to be taped, you will probably get your way if you stick to your guns and don't allow anyone to persuade you to change your mind.

The same places that will tape-record your sessions will probably want to give you a few tests. These may be intelligence tests, personality tests, or vocational tests. You should try to find out what tests are given and what those tests are supposed to measure. You have the right to ask this of the person who is testing you, and you have the right to see your score. If the agency refuses to show it to you or to explain in detail the purpose of the test you're asked to take, you've learned something important about that particular service.

Regarding a service's policies on drugs, always remember this: *You have the right to refuse to take drugs! If you feel you are being overdrugged, go somewhere else! If drugs are the only form of therapy you are to receive, go somewhere else!*

We interviewed people at approximately twenty agencies in Madison during 1971 and 1972. To include all the information we gathered would be useless to anyone not living in Madison—and in any case, much of the information is now outdated. But we have chosen information from three interviews that we think are representative of the types of services offered to women in Madison or a similar community. The first is a very large clinic associated with a university hospital. The second is a very small church-affiliated clinic, and the third is a deliberately nontraditional type of service. We would like to reemphasize that these interviews were done in 1971 and 1972. Therefore some of the information may no longer be accurate—such as numbers of women therapists, intake procedures, or other aspects of an institution that are likely to change frequently. But we include these descriptions to show an overall view of the type of information you can get *before* you walk in the front door of some service. We hope these specific interviews will encourage you to get similar information by talking to people, making phone calls, asking questions, and learning everything you can—before you put your mind in the care of any service.

PSYCHIATRIC OUT-PATIENT CLINIC, UNIVERSITY HOSPITALS*

Address: 1300 University Avenue, Madison, Wisconsin
Phone No.: (608) 262-3627

*Information based on interviews conducted in 1972.

Hours: 8:00 A.M. to 5:00 P.M. weekdays. Emergency service available 24 hours at the emergency room of the University Hospital. This is the same emergency service as for the *In-Patient* war (262-2398).

General Description: This clinic, attached to a hospital and a psychiatric training program, is quite large in both the numbers of staff and people coming in for help. Although it is attached to the university and its consumers are predominantly students, its services are available to anyone. Therapists are mainly psychiatric residents who work under the supervision of faculty in the Psychiatry Department and a number of therapists in the community who are loosely associated with the clinic. A wide variety of types of therapy are available: individual, couple, group, family, marriage counseling, etc. The clinic does not associate itself with any one school of therapy, and the director asserted that a variety of techniques were used in keeping with the "eclectic" nature of the clinic.

Finding Help

Getting an Appointment. Call the clinic and ask for an appointment. You may see somebody that afternoon. If not, you won't have to wait more than a week. The clinic is run each day by separate teams of therapists (the Monday team, the Tuesday team, etc.). During the busiest times of the year (mid-October to early May), there are up to four teams. The number of teams varies with the demand. The team on duty the first day after you call will be the team you will see.

Initial Visit. Your first visit is complicated and probably a little confusing. You spend most of the afternoon at the clinic. Here's what happens: (1) You fill out a form with your name, address, phone number, and a very brief statement of your problem. (2) You choose whether you want to talk to a single therapist or be in a group for your first day. (3) If you choose the group, you meet for about 45 minutes with other people who came to the clinic that day—you all talk with co-therapists about what to expect from the clinic, about your problems, etc. (4) If you want the privacy of a single therapist, you talk for a little while about the same things. (5) You wait around while the team of therapists meets to decide what recommendation they should make for you. (6) Then you go off with one therapist for a 45-minute interview in which the therapist gives you his or her recommendations. You probably talk more about your problems, needs, and expectations from therapy. You are asked to decide whether you want group or individual therapy. The therapist may tell you the team wants you to be in the "medication clinic" (which means you will meet with a group of people they have put on drugs as the *only* form of therapy in addition to group meetings). He or she may suggest you go into the "partial care" or "full-term care" ward of the psychiatric in-patient wards of the hospital. The clinic can legally commit you on this visit, but they say they don't without "convincing" you first. The therapist may suggest that you go to the student counseling center (which counsels academically related problems), the psychology clinic (if your problem seems applicable to behavior modification techniques), or to a private psychiatrist. The director of the clinic told us that the therapists "like to stand on their recommendations," but if you disagree with what they want you to do, you should be firm about what you want. If, for example, you don't want to go on drugs, say so immediately. They may, however, refuse to see you at all if you don't follow their "recommendations." If you have any specific requests, like wanting a woman therapist, or a particular therapist by name, *say so on this first day* at the clinic because they make it very difficult for you to change what they set up for you.

Assignment of Your Therapist: After you talk with a therapist privately or meet in a group on that first day, the whole team of therapists meets and pools information on everyone who came for help. They assign you to a therapist or a group. They try to match you with a therapist who is particularly suited to treat your problem. At this point, therapists are supposed to declare whether they feel certain problems are not in their range (one therapist we interviewed, for example, said she couldn't take a lesbian because her own feelings are too mixed up on this subject). Assignments to groups are often done by problem rather than at random. If you have been to the clinic before, they might assign you to your original therapist. If you have any specific requests— such as wanting a woman therapist or group therapy, say so *before* the team meets to make assignments, because they don't like to change their recommendations.

If You Don't Like Your Therapist. You can go through the intake procedure again or just request another therapist, but you'll have to confront your old therapist with your reasons for changing. The director told us that he understood that sometimes "two people just don't hit it off," and in this case a change was justifiable. He did not mention sexist biases of a therapist as a possible reason for change.

If They Can't Help You, Where Do They Send You? Student counseling center, psychology clinic, Dane County Mental Health Center (a public mental health facility), private psychiatrist.

Cost, Eligibility, and Length of Therapy

Cost. Initial interview costs $4.00 (free for students). The cost of following therapy sessions is negotiated by you and your therapist on a sliding scale that ranges from $2 to $30 for each session. The $2 charge can be waived. Six dollars per session is the average cost.*

Eligibility. Therapy's open to anybody. During the school year, however, 80 percent of the people in therapy are students.

*Here, as elsewhere, figures may have changed since 1972.

Length of Therapy. The clinic sees itself as providing short-term therapy (six to ten weeks) for well-defined problems. People wanting long-term therapy are often referred elsewhere. But they make exceptions—you are not obliged to stop therapy after ten weeks.

Therapists and Staff

Therapists and Staff: Four types of people are involved in the clinic: (1) faculty of psychiatry department—nineteen people (three women, sixteen men) have supervisory roles in the clinic in addition to their teaching and private practice; (2) clinical faculty members—about sixty therapists, mostly private psychiatrists or psychologists from Madison (seven or eight women, the rest men) do some therapy at the clinic; (3) residents in the psychiatry department—about forty-eight (four women as of fall '72) do most of the therapy at the clinic in their second year of residency; (4) miscellaneous—two social workers (one woman) supervise four women social work students; three graduate students in Psychiatric Nursing (women) and one woman faculty member in psychiatric nursing. These figures change often.

Training and Degrees. (1) psychiatry faculty—fourteen psychiatrists, five are clinical psychologists; (2) clinical faculty —mostly private psychiatrists; (3) residents—all have M.D.'s; (4) various people with degrees in social work, psychology, and psychiatric nursing.

Average Therapy Time. Most senior faculty are involved about 6 hours a week. Residents do 10 to 18 hours a week. For others, the load varies.

Supervision of Trainees. Each resident has three supervisors with whom he or she meets once a week.

People in Therapy. The ratio of women to men is about 50–50. At the busiest time of the year, there are sometimes as many as fifty new people a week coming to the clinic. At slow times, as few as two per week come in. Most are students.

Kinds of Therapy

Individual Therapy.   This is available, but you must ask for it on the first day. If you are in group therapy and then want to switch to individual, you can insist on a change, but you must confront your old therapist. Individual therapy sessions usually last an hour once a week, but you can meet more often if you want.

Group Therapy.   Groups usually have eight to twelve people with two co-therapists, and meet once a week for an hour. They try to assign you to a group suited to your problem. For example, one group of people may be on drug therapy, one group may consist of shy people who have trouble relating to the opposite sex, and one group may have people who are concentrating on interpersonal relationships. There are no all-women groups. The clinic has a group pool card case with your name and basic problem; this is used to form new groups. Length of the group meetings vary.

Marriage Counseling.   This is available.

Family Therapy.   This is available.

Other Group Therapy.   Counsel is available for couples who live together, including gay couples.

Association with Schools of Therapy.   This service is not associated with a particular kind of therapy. But it is well to remember that most of the therapists are residents in psychiatry. Some behavior therapy is used.

Files and Confidentiality

The clinic's *stated policy* is given here. The actual practice is unknown.

Your File. It contains mostly reports written by your therapists at various intervals. If he or she makes running notes on each session, these do not go in the file. *But a note stating that you are in therapy is sent to the student health office, if you are a student; it is attached to your student health file.*

Access to Files. Your therapist and supervisors have access to your files. The general policy of the clinic is that your file is open to no one unless that person receives written permission from you to release the file. If any government organization or employer asks for your file, the clinic gets in touch with you. This probably means that they do not guard the fact you are in therapy—only *why* you are there.

Tapes, Tests, and Drugs

Tests. Tests are administered at the discretion of your therapists.

Tapes. Tapes are used for faculty supervision of the resident therapists. Then the tapes are reused and thus destroyed within two weeks. Videotapes are sometimes used. No tapes are used without your knowledge and you can refuse to be taped if you insist.

Drugs. Drugs are used extensively. Sometimes they are the only form of therapy you will receive.

LUTHERAN SOCIAL SERVICE AGENCY*

Address: 615 Sherman Avenue, Madison, Wisconsin
Phone No.: (608) 249-6619
Hours: 8:30 A.M. to 5:30 P.M. weekdays. No emergency service unless it's during business hours, or unless you're already seeing a therapist.

General Description: This is a small private agency funded by United Givers and the Lutheran Church. Church board members OK agency board members; there is a pastor available for those who want religious counseling. But otherwise there is no connection with the church. The agency handles general kinds of therapy, adoption, and counseling for families, couples, unwed mothers, and abortion (you are assisted in making arrangements). The agency uses transactional analysis techniques.

Finding Help

Getting an Appointment. Call for an appointment. The receptionist will put you on the phone with one of the therapists, and after you say what your general problem is, he or she will make a suggestion and make an appointment. The waiting period is usually about one week.

Initial Visit. For this visit you meet with the therapist assigned to you.

Assignment of Your Therapist. You are assigned a therapist on the basis of what you say your problem is when you phone. So if you have a preference (like a woman therapist, or group therapy), say so when you make your appointment.

*Based on interviews conducted in 1972.

If You Don't Like Your Therapist. If you ask for a change, the administrators say they will give it to you. This rarely happens, however. People usually just stop coming if they don't like their therapist. It's a very small agency and it would be hard to get a fresh start with a new therapist.

If They Can't Help You, Where Do They Send You? Various other services in Madison.

Cost, Eligibility, and Length of Therapy

Cost. Sliding scale determined by income, from $1 to $25. Sometimes fees are waived.

Eligibility. Anyone can seek help here. People come from all over, with a whole cross-section of income levels. There are many young people, only a few of whom are students.

Length of Therapy. There is no set policy. Actual practice varies quite a bit.

Therapists and Staff

Therapists and Staff. There are five staff members and a consulting psychiatrist (male) who has no contact with people who come for therapy. There are also two full-time men, one half-time woman, and two women graduate students.

Training and Degrees. The two men are social workers, the woman is a psychologist, and the two graduate students are in social work.

Average Therapy Time. The graduate students carry about eight to ten in their caseloads. Others vary, depending on the type of counseling.

Supervision of Trainees. Graduate students are responsible for their own cases, but they consult with a staff member once a week. They are free to tape sessions (with person's permission), but this is not often done.

People in Therapy. No figures are available on the number of people served. Ratio of men to women is about 50–50.

Kinds of Therapy

Individual Therapy. Usually there is a once-a-week meeting for one hour; this can be more or less.

Group Therapy. Usually there is a weekly meeting for two hours. There are four or five transactional analysis groups; also a group of young women (mostly unwed mothers) that is run by a *male* therapist. Groups are not usually formed according to problems. Some groups are open-ended, some are closed to new people.

Marriage Counseling. This is available.

Family Therapy. This is available.

Other Group Therapy. The agency says it will counsel unmarried couples and gay couples (but no gay couples have ever come to them).

Child and Adolescent Therapy. This is available.

Association with Schools of Therapy. The agency favors transactional analysis, and also does some behavior therapy, but the rest is up to the individual therapist.

Files and Confidentiality

This service's *stated policy* is given here. The actual practice is unknown.

Your File. Records are kept under your name, but they consist mostly of a statement of your problem and occasional summary progress reports. There are no weekly records. A therapist's running notes are not in your file. Tests are in your file if you have taken any.

Access to Files. Anyone in the office has access to your files. Files are not kept locked. No one else is allowed to see the file without your written consent. Whether or not the information that you are in therapy is released is up to each individual therapist. After you leave therapy, inactive files are sent to the Milwaukee office.

Tapes, Tests, and Drugs

Tests. Tests are administered, but not often. Either one therapist gives the MMPI (Minnesota Multiphasic Personality Inventory), or you are referred elsewhere for a specific test.

Tapes. Tapes are used only occasionally for supervisory reasons. Your record is erased when the tape is reused.

Drugs. No drugs are prescribed.

WOMEN'S PLACE*

Address: 1101 University Avenue
Phone No.: (608) 246-0446

*Based on interviews conducted in 1973, just as Women's Place began operations.

Hours: 7:00 P.M. to 11:00 P.M. Monday through Thursday,
Sunday 1:00 P.M. to 5:00 P.M. or by appointment.

General Description: Women's Place is a mental health collective started by a group of women in Madison to offer an
alternative to traditional forms of psychotherapy. The women
in this collective feel that most therapists and schools of therapy view a woman's potential as bounded by traditional sex
roles. Women's Place is staffed primarily by lay women who
go through a training period (about ten weeks). It offers group
and individual therapy, "hot-line" telephone service, referral
services, and connections with women's groups, the Rape
Crisis Center and Gay Counseling in Madison.

Finding Help

Getting an Appointment.   No appointment is needed.
Women's Place encourages any woman to come and share
her feelings, problems, or crisis situations with members of
the collective.

Initial Visit.   You can speak with two or more women,
or you can request someone alone. These women will discuss
with you how your needs can best be met by Women's Place.

Assignment of Your Therapist.   The decision about the
type of therapy and the persons to be involved is made collectively—with you and with the other women in the collective. The emphasis is on helping *you* decide what will be best
for you.

If You Don't Like Your Therapist.   You can change.

If They Can't Help You, Where Do They Send You?   They
have a list of nonsexist therapists in the area. They may refer
you to one of these therapists or to one of the service organizations in town.

Cost, Eligibility, and Length of Treatment

Cost. There is no charge, but donations are accepted.

Eligibility. Women's Place is open to any woman.

Length of Therapy. There is a wide range of times. Some counseling is a one-time discussion; other therapy is left open-ended.

Therapists and Staff

Therapists. The women doing counseling are predominantly lay women or women who are graduate students in counseling, psychology, or social work.

Training and Degrees. No background in therapy is required, but all women must go through a training program at Women's Place. Feminist therapists in Madison often lend their expertise by giving talks or advice to counselors. The counselors work on a volunteer basis.

Average Therapy Time. This varies too much for accurate generalization.

Women in Therapy. Although Women's Place is housed near the university campus and many members of the collective are (or have been) students, it aims to reach a broad community of women. Women who come tend to be a mixture of students and women from Dane County.

Kinds of Therapy

Individual Therapy. This is available.

Group Therapy. Groups are encouraged. Members of the collective facilitate and help lead a variety of groups from CR

177

groups and study groups to therapy groups formed on the basis of specific needs.

Association with Schools of Therapy. They do not "advertise" themselves as a proponent of any one school of therapy, but they have worked out a clear theoretical perspective that forms the foundation of their collective and training program. The collective was started by women who themselves felt the limitations and contradictions of traditional therapy either through their own experience with a therapist or by their own training in mental health. Strongly influenced by the women's movement, they recognize the significance of traditional sex roles and concepts of "masculinity" and "femininity" in the origin of women's problems. They want to avoid adjusting women to their "place" in society. In terms of process, the collective wants to do away with the "God-like" power of the therapist who sees his or her "patients" on a one-to-one basis for only one hour a week. They believe that this hierarchical situation fosters dependence rather than independence. The members also feel that most therapists charge outrageous fees that effectively exclude many women from much-needed help. To break from these practices, the collective makes its organizational decisions collectively and encourages women to decide how *they* want their therapy set up.

Files and Confidentiality

Women's Place's stated policy is given here. The actual practice is unknown.

Your File. They don't have files.

Access to Files. Not applicable.

Tapes, Tests, and Drugs

Tests. They are not given.

Tapes. They are not used.

Drugs. They are not prescribed.

POSTSCRIPT*

Since several years have elapsed since we first interviewed people at these three organizations, we returned to two of them to see just how out-of-date our information had become. At the Psychiatric Out-Patient Clinic at University Hospitals, the intake procedure has been revised. More significantly, the number of women residents doing therapy has gone up to about one-third the total number of residents. The increase in women in training and women on the faculty has resulted in a lot of consciousness-raising and a new sensitivity to women's issues. The clinic now regularly makes various kinds of therapy available for groups of women; it also works closely with campus police to provide immediate help for any rape victim who reports the assault to the police.

At this writing, Women's Place has been offering lay counseling to women for several years. The collective is administered on a volunteer basis by three rotating coordinators and several committees (training committee, funding committee, in-service committee, etc.). At any given time, there are about fifteen women who serve as staffers one or two evenings a week. These women go through a ten- to twelve-week training program run by staffers for three hours a week. Modeled on "empathy training," the emphasis is on teaching "listening" skills, "reflecting" skills, and "group facilitator"

*Based on follow-up interviews conducted in 1977.

179

skills. Prospective staffers are asked to pay a small fee for their training and to make a one-year commitment to do counseling on a volunteer basis at Women's Place. "Consciousness raising" on feminist issues is not formally structured into the training; instead, it is assumed that anyone volunteering that amount of time would not advocate traditional roles for women. Training continues for all staffers through a once-a-month in-service workshop. Programs vary all the way from a professional therapist to someone from the Rape Crisis Center. Since no one is paid and the group pays no rent (space is donated by a church), expenses are low. Benefit dinners and fees for training have raised enough money for publicity and phone bills. Currently, the collective is writing a grant proposal. The rapid turnover rate of staffers is a problem and the administrative load is heavy.

Women's Place gets about fifty phone calls a month and five "walk-ins" a week. Half of the women come in once or twice; half return for about three months of counseliing. In spite of its location near the campus, most women are not students; most are in the 30 to 40 age range.

Women and Mental Institutions: Some Issues

With our focus on "out-patient" therapy for women, a whole area of psychological services for women hasn't been touched upon in this book as yet—mental institutions. Various books and articles on mental institutions, however, convinced us that it would be a serious gap in a guide to women and therapy to exclude some consideration of "in-patient" care. In particular, Phyllis Chesler's *Women and Madness*, Phil Brown's anthology *Radical Psychology*, Thomas S. Szasz's *Ideology and Insanity*, D. L. Rosenhan's study, "On Being Sane in Insane Places," and the journal *Rough Times* (formerly *The Radical Therapist* and currently *State and Mind*) provided a framework of analysis and information that allowed us to interview a number of women who had been in mental institutions. We quickly learned how vast and complex the subject is. To describe fully what women have experienced in mental institutions and to provide a complete guide for women in hospitals would certainly take a whole book—one that could be more knowledgeably and forcefully written by women who have been in mental institutions. But because we could not ignore this larger dimension of women's suffering in therapy, we have written this chapter to provide an introduction to the central issues. It is by no means a definitive statement about women in mental institutions, but it should clarify the questions you need to ask and direct you to sources that can offer more complete information.

Most of the material in this book is as applicable to women in institutions as it is to those on the outside. But the forms of oppression that exist in out-patient therapy are many times worse for women who have to live under the control of a hospital staff twenty-four hours a day. The power of the psychiatrists, nursing staff and attendants, and the damage that can be done by their preconceptions of women, are multiplied—first because in a mental institution women spend more time as "patients" and second because in an institution the doctors and the staff are freer to use more forceful and destructive techniques, methods, or pressures to achieve their goals. No matter how good the intentions of the staff are, the ultimate weapon held over every patient's head is the fact that the people who set up or enforce the rules and control everyday life are the same people who determine standards of "sanity" and "insanity." Those on the staff whom patients may resent and fear are the very people who hold the power to release the patients with their official stamp of "sanity."

One ex-patient reported that mental institutions represent "the Patriarchy written large." The judges who commit a person, the husbands who sign the papers, the administrators of the hospital, and the psychiatrists and other staff are almost always men. The nurses often have quite a lot of immediate control over patients because the doctors rarely have much contact with those who are confined in the mental institution. Many nurses wield this power very harshly (like Big Nurse in Ken Kesey's *One Flew Over the Cuckoo's Nest*)—perhaps because they've managed to make a small place for themselves in a man's world. To exercise and maintain their station, they can be harder on women patients than even the male doctors. The same ex-patient told us that the description of the power exercised over the patients in Kesey's book was no exaggeration. But Kesey's point that women like Big Nurse rule the hospital, and even the male doctors, is wrong. No matter how much control the nurses have through daily contact, mental hospitals are not "matriarchies"; they are male-dominated institutions.

But it's not only the fact that the people who run the hospitals are men that causes problems for women—women judges and psychiatrists have sometimes been as hard on women as have their male colleagues. Inside most hospitals, the idea of what's "normal," "healthy" behavior for a woman is a highly intensified version of the conventional norms on the outside. Most women in this country today, for example, wear makeup and spend enormous amounts of money, time, and energy on their wardrobes. But if we on the "outside" want to wear pants or go without makeup, we can find friends who share our values. Inside many mental hospitals, women are rewarded if they exhibit stereotypic "feminine" behavior. If they refuse to act or look "feminine," certain privileges can be withheld or withdrawn.

For example, one ex-patient told us:

> *On my ward the staff always noticed if you "fixed yourself up." When I appeared in hair curlers one day, I was given a weekend pass. A friend of mine was told she could apply for an outside job if she would wear a skirt and put on makeup.*

Women who choose a lifestyle that doesn't "fit" the cultural ideas of women's roles have a hard enough time in the everyday world—but they suffer more within a mental institution. For example, lesbians on the outside certainly have a rough time facing people's prejudices and hate. But today it is possible for them to find women who are not threatened by what they are. Inside a hospital the distaste of the culture for lesbians is multiplied—a lesbian is usually considered to be "sick" and she is constantly reminded by the staff of her sexual "craziness." Women who wear pants, who refuse makeup or curlers, or who assert their opinions strongly are much more apt to be accused of being lesbians or latent lesbians than similar women on the outside. One ex-patient told us: "In one of the hospitals I was in, the lesbian in my ward was given a lobotomy. She believed that the lobotomy was performed to "cure" what the staff saw as her "sexual deviance."

In our culture, single women and women who don't want children or who get divorced are thought not to fulfill the ideal of womanhood, but there is usually some subculture in which they can find a comfortable place. But in the mental hospital the stereotypes for women and the roles thought to be "proper" for them are even more rigidly defined. Women in an institution are often taught that they must conform to the norms. Their refusal is interpreted as a sign that they are still "crazy" and should not be released until they learn to be smoothly functioning "women." If you on the outside believe that your therapist has ideas about women's roles that are too restrictive for you, you can get up your courage and quit—even though it may be hard to have this much faith in yourself, you *can* do it. But a woman in a mental hospital cannot walk out those doors until she convinces the *staff* she is sane. And since "sane" for a woman all too often means willing acceptance of a traditional "feminine" role, she must conform in order to get out. Mental institutions, even more than out-patient therapy situations, are instruments that attempt to adjust and socialize women to an unjust society. In the words of an ex–mental patient:

> I was divorced from my husband and had custody of my child. I went into a mental hospital after my ex-husband kidnapped my child. They were always telling me to go back to my husband. And other women, too—go back and be good wives and mothers, that was the message. The staff was consciously setting out to socialize me and other women into accepting a domestic role happily. As for the men patients, the staff worked to get them to function as workers and breadwinners.

Another ex-patient said that mental hospitals are "warehouses for the poor," the "last frontier" where those who don't fit in can be stored. One of the greatest misconceptions about mental hospitals, she told us, is the belief that there is much therapy taking place in them. This certainly varies from institution to institution, but on the whole *very little therapy, and almost no individual therapy*, is done in mental hospitals.[1] Wards often have daily group sessions or meetings, but many patients are never assigned an individual therapist. Patients are often overwhelmed with the reality that there is little attempt in a hospital to work on their problems; most of the energy is spent on getting them to adjust to the hospital community. One ex-patient of a university hospital in-patient ward said:

> *All the rules they set up and the things they rewarded you for were aimed at getting you to relate nicely with other patients instead of helping you work on the problems you needed to face in order to get along in the outside world. For example, I wanted to get a pass to go to my class. I was told I could go if I could get two other patients to agree that I should go. Most of the other patients were so involved with their own suffering that I couldn't get through to them.*

The shortage of therapists is probably most true at large and/or public institutions. Medical hospitals often have one or two wards for mental patients, and in these smaller places you may have a better chance of getting help. But not always. One woman who admitted herself to an inpatient psychiatric ward of a hospital told us of her stay:

> *I saw a therapist when I was admitted and when I was discharged. That was it. I had a sort of group therapy once a day. The closest thing they had to group therapy was a meeting every morning. They went around the circle of people and each "patient" bared her soul. If she didn't, social pressure and recollections of embarrassing situations were put on her—like getting confronted with your suicide attempts, past "hysterical" behavior, etc. Everyone was writing down what you said. Tensions were unbearably high and many people were kept calm only because of the solidarity among the patients.*

Often, if you get a therapist at all, it is because a doctor has decided to single you out and work on your case—maybe because your "illness" is more "interesting" or "rare." This can cause a barrier between you and the other patients, because they will envy your special treatment.

But emphasizing the lack of therapists in most mental institutions isn't to suggest that simply finding a hospital with a better staff/patient ratio is the answer for anyone desperately seeking help. In one ex-patient's words:

> *The shortage of therapists is not the problem so much as what kind of therapy is possible in a mental institution. Even in hospitals where there is enough staff to hold group therapy, patients know they must hide their real feelings and say only what is considered "normal." Group therapy—and individual therapy—behind the walls of an institution is just another occasion where patients have to conform to the hospital's version of sanity. Attendance at group therapy is most often mandatory. Patients are punished for not attending by having "privileges" (visitors, letters, phone calls, a walk on the grounds) denied, and their hospital stay prolonged. It is questionable whether surrounding patients with highly trained professionals who hold the values of the dominant society is going to do the patients any good. Patients do need people to talk to—and to a large extent patients have each other—but simply improving the staff/patient ratio is not the answer.*

So it isn't a therapist you need to deal with in a mental hospital as much as it is the whole hospital staff—the attendants, the nurses, sometimes social workers, committees of psychiatrists, and hospital administrators. And once you cross that hospital threshold to become a "patient," you are likely to lose your credibility, your validity, your whole identity in the eyes of most staff members. You are the "crazy," "sick" one and therefore everything you say is doubted.

A woman who had worked in a mental hospital said:

> *I liked one patient in particular and was moved and upset by his account of what had happened to him before he came to the hospital—how he had not received credit for some special job he had done. I asked the doctor about the man and the doctor told me directly: "Don't*

pay too much attention to the old man. You can't believe anything he says." I felt confused by the doctor's advice because I thought there was a chance that the patient could have been telling the story accurately; but I figured that the doctor knew better than I could how to understand "crazy" people and so I gradually dismissed everything the patient told me. Now, in recalling this incident years later, I wonder how it must have felt to be believed by nobody. Bad enough to drive anybody crazy, I suppose.

The impact of continuously not being believed can be devastating, especially for women, for it reinforces the self-doubt, self-hatred, and self-blame that is a part of most women's problems. Even women on the outside fight passivity, dependency, self-hatred, and the sense of having no identity. But this is intensified inside the hospital. When everyone doubts your credibility, the insecurity and uncertain sense of self common to many women becomes a total negation of identity. Women patients often come to accept what the staff thinks of them. Furthermore, dependency and passivity are encouraged by the whole hospital setup. In many institutions, every moment of a patient's day is planned—most wards don't allow you to make even the smallest decisions about daily life (what to eat, what to wear, where to go, etc.). Angry and aggressive behavior is often expected of a male patient, but when a woman expresses anger, she is more likely to be immediately punished with some drug, seclusion, or even beating, according to Chesler.[2]

Formal contact with staff members is often hostile and humiliating. "They put you on the defensive; they use a lot of pressure to see if you will crack," one ex-patient told us as she explained that the staff is seldom supportive. A practice that seems to institutionalize this kind of attack goes under various names, but is often known among staff members as a "stress interview" (for patients, the staff calls it a "patient presentation") at which a patient must face a large group of questioners who theoretically attempt to reveal her problems by putting her in an unbearably stressful situation. The result is often the destruction of the last shreds of self-confidence.

One woman described her first "stress interview" to us:

I was transferred from one state mental hospital to another. On my first day, I had to join the line in a hot stuffy hall of people waiting for their "patient presentation" or "stress interview." After two hours of watching other patients emerge from the examining room shaken, frightened, and often crying, it was my turn. I entered determined to remain cool and self-controlled. I faced a doctor sitting at the end of a long table by himself. The staff was lined up behind him—mostly nurses, probably in training, since this "interview" is used as a teaching technique to demonstrate how patients react to "stress." I sat down without being asked—an aggressive act.

"Are you married?"
"No."
"Why not?"
"I don't feel a need to be."
"Have you had any boyfriends?"
"I've had my share."
"Are you still friends with them?"
"Some of them."
"That's your problem—you're too friendly. Has your doctor prescribed any drugs?"
"Fiorinal."
"What's in it?"
"I'm not sure."
The doctor turned to his staff, waved his hand like a conductor, and the women all repeated in unison: "Fiorinal is nothing but a bona fide aspirin."

This woman and two other ex-patients explained that "stress interviews" and other examinations of women often begin right off with questions about their sexual life. Like sex objects, women are immediately defined and categorized in terms of their sexual relationships with men. Yet ironically, celibacy is demanded in the institution, even on co-ed wards. The double standard about sex for unmarried men and women is also sometimes strong—as these words of a former patient illustrate:

When I was committed to a mental hospital, I was worried that I might be pregnant. After I had been there a few days, I hoped that they would be lenient and helpful or "progressive" about an un-married woman, and so I asked for a pregnancy test. I got my preg-nancy test, but the staff immediately categorized me as a "loose woman" and seldom missed a chance to make cutting comments about my sex life. When I would have a male visitor, for example, they would ask me if he was "the one."

In response to staff hostility or distance, patients often band together for support. A former patient told us:

There is an immediate bond among patients. Their common suffering brings them together—united against the staff, the powers that control their daily lives and pass on their sanity so that they can get out.

The destruction of identity and self-confidence that is so common in mental hospitals makes it very hard for women to make it on their own once they are released. In the first place, coming out of an institution induces genuine culture shock— you have to get on buses, in cars; you have to buy your clothes, your food, deal with shopkeepers; you have to make countless daily decisions, and so forth. But the feeling of confusion and fear which ought to be understood as normal for such a change is often felt by recent ex-patients as evidence that they are still "crazy"—that they should go back to the hospital. One ex-patient said:

When I finally walked down the sidewalk on the outside of the hospital walls, I felt a sinking, lonely fear in the face of an empty future in which I would have to decide what to do with my life. Feeling this fear convinced me that I must still be crazy, and I almost walked right back into the hospital.

Little is done in most mental hospitals to give women the self-confidence to believe that they *can* be independent.

When I got out of the hospital I was terrified at the thought of riding the MBTA in Boston—had the price gone up? Could I get change? I finally told someone I was from out of town and asked about the fare.

Economically and legally, there are likely to be problems for women coming out—no credit cards or credit for a loan, difficulty in getting a job, problems with custody of children, with getting a driver's license, or regular health insurance.

David Rosenhan's study, reported in his article "On Being Sane in Insane Places," summarizes and confirms our general observations on the difficulties mental patients face. His work is not focused specifically on women patients, but his conclusions about the misdiagnoses and depersonalization of both male and female patients provide a useful description of the general conditions in mental institutions that are then compounded by sexism. Rosenhan, a Stanford professor, set up an experiment in which "eight sane people gained secret admission" to twelve different mental institutions on the east and west coasts.[3] His purpose was to determine the accuracy of psychiatric diagnosis and to observe conditions in mental hospitals without the staffs' knowledge. The eight pseudo-patients (he himself was the first to be admitted) told the people in the admissions office that they were "hearing voices"; but after admission, all patients answered every question truthfully and claimed (or exhibited) no "symptoms" of any kind. They were cooperative with the staff and obedient to all instructions—with the one exception that they did not consume the 2,100 pills they were given in a period of time that averaged 19 days. The diagnosis at the various hospitals (with one exception) was "schizophrenia," and they were discharged with the diagnosis "schizophrenia in remission," *not* a formal statement of "sanity."

In a follow-up study, Rosenhan arranged another experiment with a teaching and research hospital. The staff was told that at some time in the following three months, one or more pseudopatients would attempt to be admitted to the hospital. Various staff members (psychiatrists, nurses, attendants, etc.) identified up to *forty-one* patients as pseudopatients (out of a total of 193). But Rosenhan had arranged for the admission of *no* pseudopatients. On the basis of these two studies, Rosenhan concludes in his article that there is little scientific reliability to psychiatric diagnosis. This phenomena of "massive errors" in labeling people "mentally ill" or "insane" has serious consequences for both patients and ex-patients. Unlike most medical diagnoses, psychiatric diagnoses "carry with them personal, legal, and social stigmas." And equally important, the psychiatric "tag" of illness colors everyone's perceptions of the patients' behavior. He argues that if any of the staff see a person as "sane," that category makes them perceive such feelings as occasional anger or depression as a "normal" part of life. But when the same person is labeled "insane," "schizophrenic," "manic-depressive," or "crazy" (etc.), then those feelings are viewed as symptoms of mental illness. He concludes: "As far as I can determine, diagnoses were in no way affected by the relative health of the circumstances of a pseudopatient's life. Rather, the reverse occurred: The perception of his circumstances was shaped entirely by the diagnosis." In other words, the label of insanity invalidates the feelings and ideas of a patient in the eyes of many staff members.

Rosenhan understands the potential of such labeling to destroy the identity and dignity of people in mental hospitals. The general conditions that he and his pseudopatients observed (and experienced) as patients compounded the destructiveness of psychiatric labeling. In a variety of ways, the hospital environment dehumanizes and depersonalizes the patients and imbues them with a sense of powerlessness. As the first aspect of depersonalization, Rosenhan notes that there is not only little "therapy" done, but the patient–staff interactions are minimal. What exists is mainly custodial. Staff spend most of their time on duty inside a "glass cage," separated from the patients. They emerge to give medications, fold laundry, watch TV, etc. In the hospitals they studied, for example, attendants spent an average of 11.3 percent of their time outside the cage; day-time nurses came out of the cage on the average of 11.5 times per shift. Psychiatrists appeared on the ward 6.7 times per day. The higher a person's position on the hospital hierarchy was, the less time he or she spent with patients.

Secondly, the staff continually avoided contacts initiated by patients as if they too shared the common attitudes toward mental illness—"fear, hostility, aloofness, suspicion and dread." While Rosenhan stresses that staff avoidance seldom originates in outright "malice" or "stupidity," he argues that the hospital environment (especially with its psychological and physical segregation of patients and staff) reinforces this process of dehumanization. Questions that pseudopatients and real patients asked were often ignored, answered quickly without eye contact (or with head averted), or greeted with non sequiturs. For example,

> The encounter frequently took the following bizarre form: (pseudo-patient) "Pardon me, Dr. X. Could you tell me when I am eligible for grounds privileges?" (physician) "Good morning, Dave. How are you today?" (Moves off without waiting for a response.)

Depersonalization also took more brutal forms:

> I have records of patients who were beaten by staff for the sin of having initiated verbal contact. During my own experience, for example, one patient was beaten in the presence of other patients for having approached an attendant and told him, "I like you." Occasionally, punishment meted out to patients for misdemeanors seemed so excessive that it could not be justified by the most radical interpretations of psychiatric canon.

While abusive treatment was common, it mostly occurred when only one staff member was present with one or more patients. The abuse often ceased when another staff member approached because "staff are credible witnesses. Patients are not." Rosenhan concludes that the hospital environment makes patients invisible nonpersons without credibility in the eyes of the staff. This experience of depersonalization, compounded by a loss of civil rights and privacy adds up to a condition of "powerlessness" so severe that it is enough to drive anyone "crazy."

Recognition of the grave psychological dangers Rosenhan describes is not in itself sufficient protection if you are on your way to a mental hospital. You should have some concrete information on issues relating to the existing conditions of mental hospitals. Especially since the laws vary from state to state and the kinds of treatments and conditions in mental hospitals vary from institution to institution, we can only point to the areas of difficulty and outright danger in mental institutions. In the following sections we can give you some ideas of the *questions* to ask, and the *issues* involved—not all the answers.

LEGAL ISSUES

If you think you might ever go—either willingly or un-willingly—to a mental institution, it is absolutely critical that you find out what the laws in your state have to say about the rights and status of mental patients. There are a number of legal issues you should find out about—everything from your property rights to your rights to refuse such "treatment" as lobotomy, sterilization, or electroshock therapy. The most important legal issues you should investigate are the laws about commitment, voluntary admission, and release.

Commitment

"Commitment" is a legal term meaning you must go to a mental institution and you cannot leave the hospital until you are declared sane by professionals. Find out in your state who can commit you. It can be a lawyer, doctor, psychiatrist, judge, policeman, husband, parents, and children in varying combinations and numbers depending entirely on your state laws. Your age is no protection. Women who resist the limitations of the socially acceptable, the restrictions of the tradi-tional "feminine role," or the outright use of power by a man close to her are all too often unjustly committed by doctors who readily side with the males in the family.

Many people—therapists and psychiatrists as well as ex-patients—believe that commitment plays an extensive social function that goes far beyond the supposed rehabilitation of a clearly pathological person. For those criminally committed (sometimes for indefinite "sentences" that would exceed a stay in prison), mental institutions have become an extension of the penal system.[4] This has been especially true for men. In many mental hospitals treating alcoholism, for example, many men are in the program as an alternative to prison. For women, however, commitment has mainly functioned as an instrument of the status quo rather than as an alternative to a prison sentence. Women alcoholics are frequently committed by their families. Commitment is in many cases an institutional tool by which husbands can extend their control over the fate of their wives.

Following is a series of observations concerning the involuntary commitment of women to mental institutions—all related to us by ex-patients:

> *After a woman in the hospital began to trust me, she told me the story of how she had been committed. Her husband wanted intercourse every night of the week; she didn't want sex so often and felt two times a week was enough. The examining psychiatrist agreed with the husband that something must be wrong with her.*

> *I was awakened one morning by the police with commitment papers. My parents, upset by my activities in the anti-war movement, had found a psychiatrist who agreed that I should be committed. I was released after three heavily drugged months during which I wore makeup, kept my anger hidden, and acted submissive so as to convince the staff of my sanity.*

> *At the hospital, I met a woman who had been beaten and finally committed by her husband. She admitted to me that her husband had made her put on boxing gloves before they went to bed. Here's where the label "crazy" can hurt so much. The doctor could say "Don't pay any attention to what she says—she's paranoid." Once she has been labeled delusion-ridden, no one has to believe her story and her commitment is justified or rationalized by this circular reasoning in the minds of the experts.*

> *I met a woman at the hospital whose husband used to beat her regularly. In desperation, she finally swallowed enough pills to kill herself. Her husband took her to the hospital, where the doctors recommended commitment. After she recovered, she began to tell everybody she didn't*

need to be in an institution—her husband had driven her to suicide by his beatings. They didn't believe her, but agreed to ask the husband if what she said was true. The husband, frightened by the seriousness of her suicide attempt, admitted that everything she had said was correct. On the grace of his honesty alone, she was released. How many more women are in mental institutions today because their husbands could so easily escape blame by saying that their wives had "made everything up?"

Phyllis Chesler quoted a woman she interviewed:

After my husband left me and the baby, I was too depressed to do anything. I was a twenty-year-old mother, and back home dependent on my parents. . . . I didn't go to college because my mother didn't think I was smart enough. My father was very violent to me. . . . It was a shitty family and I escaped it by getting married. . . . So I came back home and said, "I'm home," and my mother said, "Like hell you are. You made your bed, lie in it." So I had to threaten that I'd kill myself . . . and my mother said, "Okay, if you're crazy you belong in a hospital. . . ." My father knew the director of this private loony bin and they all told me to sign myself in and be grateful.[5]

Susan Dworkin Levering tells of yet another woman committed against her will:

Linda is in her late thirties. Her husband had her committed after she left him and filed for divorce. At her commitment hearing, he testified that she was having a "fantasy love affair" or hallucinating. She had in fact fallen in love with another man, with whom she had not had sexual relations.[6]

Pauline Bart tells of a number of women committed to mental institutions because of "depression" that has painfully arisen out of their inability to deal with the sense of emptiness and uselessness occurring in middle age, when they no longer feel needed by husband or children.[7]

Voluntary Admission

"Voluntary admission" is a term used to describe a person's own decision to commit him/herself to a mental hospital. A person's status, treatment, and rights in a mental hospital can vary with use of the labels "commitment" or "voluntary admission." In some places, a "voluntary admission" tag can be changed to "commitment" if you "misbehave" or show signs of "craziness." But *seldom* does "voluntary admission" mean that a person can walk *out* the door anytime she wants to. If you are considering admitting yourself, *find out from a lawyer the laws in your state* about your rights to leave. Many institutions have a "preliminary thirty-day observation period"; find out what this really means for you in terms of commitment.

One woman said:

> *I did not voluntarily go to a mental hospital. But when I was committed I was offered the chance to sign a "conditional voluntary" form stating that I was admitting myself. They told me, "Either sign this paper or we'll commit you." I signed because I thought I might be able to leave when I wanted. I was wrong. I still had to be judged "sane" by doctors before I could leave. Hospitals prefer their records to show large numbers of voluntary admissions; and the national statistics on the ratio of commitments to voluntary admissions are highly distorted by the common practice of threatening patients with commitment if they don't sign the voluntary papers.*

Release

The state laws vary greatly regarding release, too. But if a person is committed, she cannot leave of her own free will. If you voluntarily admit yourself, *you may still have to convince the staff of your sanity* before you can leave. If the staff determines that you have suicidal tendencies, you can be kept in the hospital. This may have its benefits—some lives may really be saved. But others—especially those who appear "crazy" to the staff because they don't fulfill the norms—may also lose their civil rights.

Most states have various kinds of laws requiring sanity hearings to be held at certain legally set intervals (six months, one year, etc.). Judges, psychiatrists, and/or staff members may make such judgments, depending on the state. In any case, recommendations of the hospital staff would be weighed heavily. According to the reports of many ex-patients, it doesn't appear that a person is likely to be able to depend on these hearings for justice. Here are the words of three such people:

> *The hearings are a kangaroo court. They generally last 15 to 30 seconds —a rubber stamp for the hospital staff.*

> *I had been waiting eagerly for my hearing because I really thought I had a chance to get out. Two days before the hearing, I was put on an extremely heavy dosage of a depressant drug. I could barely eat, talk, or walk. I had to be helped into the hearing room by two aides because the drugs made it so hard for me to walk. I know my eyes were glassy and "crazy" looking. I couldn't talk. I saw my parents looking at me and agreeing immediately with the judge that I was not yet "ready" for the outside world. My hearing took 15 seconds.*

And a therapist said:

> *One day I was standing in the hall outside some sanity hearings. I saw a woman waiting to be led before the judge. Just before she was brought into the room, one of the attendants gave her a shot of some drug.*

Sterilization

Your consent for sterilization is *not* required in some states. If you suspect that sterilization will be "suggested" or ordered for you, find out as soon as possible what your legal rights are to control your own body. If you do not have the right to decide for yourself, then try to find out who has the authority to decide—a judge, a committee, the staff, etc.? Do you have a right to be represented by a lawyer on this issue?

If you are a minority woman, then the sterilization issue is particularly important for you. Sterilization and sterilization abuses—that is, coercive operations or withholding of accurate information—affect minority women disproportionate to their numbers in the general population. According to some statistics, 20 percent of all married Black women have been sterilized in the United States (three times the percentage of white married women). Some 33 percent of Puerto Rican women of childbearing age have been sterilized; and about 25 percent of Native American women of childbearing age have been sterilized. Sterilization procedures for the poor often include little or no provisions against abuse. Women are sometimes not told they are being sterilized, or their consent is "asked" while they are in labor. Sometimes "consent" is gained through coercion—with threats such as a cutoff of welfare funds. Many women are never informed that the operation is not reversible.[8] These abuses of the right to be informed, uncoerced consent are serious enough for minority women *outside* mental institutions. Given the high number of poor and minority women *in* mental hospitals, you would be wise to assume that sterilization abuse occurs inside the hospital as well.

Legal Aid

Check with your state laws to see whether you have a right to a lawyer—you probably do. You may really have to go to a lot of trouble to get in touch with a lawyer.

An ex-patient told us:

> In my hospital, it was hard to find a pay phone. There wasn't even any money around (you had nothing to use it for) and so getting change for a phone call was difficult. Nobody will hand you a phone and say, "Here, you have a right to call a lawyer." You may not even be told your rights.

One woman told us you probably have the right to a court-appointed lawyer in most states. But she warned that patients should not assume that a court lawyer will be a real advocate. She suggested that you try to get a Legal Aid lawyer instead. It's difficult to know how much we can generalize from her experience, but here's why she makes that recommendation:

> *After I got out of the hospital, I was trying to regain custody of my child through the courts—before I entered the hospital, my husband had kidnapped my son. The court got hold of my records from the mental institution; and so I was forced to admit that I had had an affair since my divorce—some of the details were in my file. My own* court-appointed *lawyer said that "this woman represents the downfall of America as we know and love it." This sentiment was too much for the judge, who commented that he didn't see anything "balmy" (archaic for "crazy") about me, and I was very fortunately awarded my child.*

Her distrust of court-appointed lawyers is confirmed as reasonable by Phil Brown in his outline of changes necessary for mental hospitals—he advocates lawyers, "not state hired."[9]

You should also check with a lawyer to see what the laws in your state say about your legal "competency" to handle your own financial affairs.

If you need help *finding* a lawyer, get in touch with the local Legal Aid society or with the ACLU (American Civil Liberties Union). Some useful resources on the legal rights of mental patients include the ACLU paperback *Legal Rights of Mental Patients* and the handbook called *Some Facts You Should Know About Mental Patients' Rights*, which has been written by ex-patients of the Boston Mental Patients' Liberation Front (BMPLF, P.O. Box 156, W. Somerville, Mass., 02144). The Patient Advocacy Legal Service (PALS, Washington University Law School, St. Louis, Missouri, 63130) operates as a clearinghouse for information in mental commitment areas. The Bill of Rights for Mental Patients, drawn up by members of the Mental Patients' Liberation Project as a statement of what *should* be instead of what *is*, is reprinted in Phil Brown's *Radical Psychology*. See also the "Resources" section at the end of this book for addresses of chapters of mental patients' liberation groups.

KINDS OF TREATMENT

If there is so little therapy done in mental hospitals, what kinds of "treatment" can you expect?

Drugs

Almost everyone in a mental hospital is put on drugs, often as soon as they enter. Drugs appear to be the main instrument of adjusting the patients to the hospital community so things can run smoothly. If a woman patient gets loud or aggressive, drugs may be used—often in connection with seclusion—to control and punish her (especially since aggressive behavior is not as acceptable for a woman as for a man).

One ex-patient said to us about drugs:

> Drugs are a chemical used to keep the hospital functioning by preventing you from feeling what you are feeling. Someone who hasn't had these drugs cannot imagine how powerful they are; if you have been given a depressant, it can take all of your strength to do basic, simple things like hold your head up, concentrate on something, talk, eat, or walk. All the energy that could be used in working on one's problems go into learning how to deal with those drugs.

And patients are seldom told what they are taking or why, or what possible side effects the drugs might have.

Some important questions involving drugs administered in mental institutions are: Who prescribes these drugs—someone who has talked with you and knows your situation? Can you refuse them? Can you throw them out? Who supervises their use? Why are women often kept on heavy doses of drugs after they leave therapy (an excuse for poor therapy?)? Are the abuses of prescribed drugs for women outside the mental institution just intensified inside the hospital?

In her book, Phyllis Chesler quotes a physician's words about drug usage for women with emotional problems:

> The drug industry openly acknowledges the enslavement of women, as shown in an ad with a woman behind bars made up of brooms and

200

mops. The caption reads: "You can't set her free but you can make her feel less anxious." Another one pictures a woman who, we are told, has an M.A. degree but who now must be content with the PTA and housework. This we are advised, contributes to her gynecological complaints, which should be treated with drugs.[10]

A more recent ad in a medical journal shows the smiling face of a secretary hard at work on her typewriter. "Awake on the job, yet anxieties resolved," the headline reads. The drug Tranxene® is recommended for patients with "anxiety," problems, and it promises to "calm" the anxious secretary without "compromising" her ability to work. Instead of treating the cause of her anxiety—perhaps a bad situation at work —drugs are prescribed to help her adjust more calmly to the status quo.

More questions: In exactly how many cases are drugs the only form of therapy used? What kinds of drugs are used? What is known about the long-term effects of Thorazine, Mellaril, Stelazine, Valium, Librium, Prolixin, insulin treatments? What are their side effects? Is it true that heavy doses of some of these drugs can cause serious physical problems, as some medical doctors have warned? Are these drugs in any way a cure for "mental illness" (the way penicillin is a cure for infections)? Do the drugs merely cover up all evidence of distress? Do they help people deal with their problems or make them *unable* to deal with problems?

One woman said:

> I was kept on heavy doses of Thorazine all during my stay in a mental hospital. I kept falling asleep because of the drugs, and when I fell asleep at group meetings, I was penalized for it.

One ex-patient who had had experiences in several public and private mental institutions in two states, told us she had some of the answers to our questions. She wrote:

> Drugs are prescribed by the ward doctor, who in a state hospital has several wards to take care of. He usually doesn't even see the patient

—just routinely orders something that will keep a new admission quiet. Chances are good that if you're allergic to some particular drug, no one will find out until it's too late.

Usually, you're not told what kind of drug you're getting, or if your medication is changed, why it's being changed. Persistent questioning can sometimes get the answer out of the doctor—if you ever get a chance to see him. In most hospitals, drugs are part of the "accepted" treatment and can't be openly refused by patients, although frequently patients will pretend to swallow their pills and later flush them down the toilet. Many women who come into an instituion drug-free leave the hospital drug-dependent. They think they can't get along without the pills because that's what everyone in the hospital —and their friends and families—have told them. I was so afraid of going back to the hospital that I took little yellow pills for months and months after I got out. They helped keep me working away at my clerical job, even though I was sleeping 12 and 14 hours the rest of the time. I was considered "recovered"—or, in technical terms, a paranoid schizophrenic "in remission."

Drugs are a substitute for the human contact patients need. They stop behavior that is disturbing the staff and give the appearance of normality. As long as patients look like they're OK—i.e., they get up and get dressed and get in line for meals and don't bother anyone—there is no need for the staff to recognize the real emotional state of the patients and try to extend themselves in helping patients through crises.

Seclusion

Is there a therapeutic purpose in "seclusion"? The fact is that it is a very frequent form of "treatment" in mental hospitals.

Three ex-patients, with experience in six hospitals, described seclusion to us:

You are locked in a bare room with absolutely nothing to do—sometimes for days at a time. The lights are on 24 hours a day. No one is allowed to talk to you. When you want to go to the bathroom, you have to bang on the door until an attendant comes to get you. In one hospital, two patients died in seclusion.

Seclusion is often used, like drugs, for punitive purposes —to keep the hospital running smoothly. One ex-patient said:

> *I saw a woman start to cry in the lounge of her ward. She was given a shot and thrown into seclusion for a couple of days—to "quiet her."*

Another woman said:

> *I was brought into the hospital on a stretcher. I was crying. They put me immediately into seclusion for four days.*

Aversive Therapy

Aversive therapy is a behaviorist method of conditioning a person to hate or have a violent reaction against something she or he formerly liked. For example, some behaviorist therapists have attempted to "treat" homosexuals by conditioning them to feel nausea at the sight of the naked body of someone of the same sex. Aversive therapy is done through the use of electroshock, nausea drugs, loud noise, or any unpleasant stimulus. It is meant to be painful—in fact, it has to be painful to work.[11] But this kind of treatment raises serious questions: Who decides that aversive therapy is what a patient in a mental institution needs? Does a patient have any choice in the matter? Let's say you are satisfied with being lesbian—are you faced with a choice of aversive therapy or a longer stay in the hospital? Is this technique primarily used on poor people? middle-class people? What types of problems is it primarily used for—drug addiction, alcoholism, homosexuality, "deviant" sexual behavior? Is it permanently harmful? Does it work? Are patients told they will receive aversive therapy? Are they told about possible side effects?

A psychology intern student had this to say about a drug used in aversive therapy:

> *One nausea drug, Antabuse, causes a person to become violently ill for several hours after any intake of alcohol. People in the program where I work were only told that it would be "unpleasant" to drink alcohol. They drank and some said later they thought they were dying.*

The Token Economy System

A "token economy" in a mental institution is considered a form of "treatment." This is a behavior modification system by which people in institutions must earn tokens that buy "privileges" (sometimes even room and board). It is becoming increasingly popular in many hospitals. In the token system, tokens are earned by behavior the staff considers socially acceptable. The system is intended to be therapeutic because it tangibly rewards patients for acting "normal" and "conditions" them to change their behavior. But what is rewarded is necessarily the behavior consistent with the values of the staff. And "proper" behavior for a woman patient all too frequently involves the traditionally "feminine" qualities and duties surrounding dress, domestic chores, language, manners, passivity, and so forth. To get her privileges (and sometimes even her meals), a woman may have to conform to traditional prejudices.

Susan Dworkin Levering wrote about the use of the token economy system alone.

> To earn tokens, [the patient] can change her underwear, make the beds in the men's ward, cut up rags for rag rugs, perform janitorial tasks or wear a girdle. Her girdle has to be new, however—an old one won't entitle her to a token. Sometimes patients are given special rewards of a visit to the ward beauty parlor.[12]

Important questions remain: Can a patient decide whether or not she *wants* to go on a token economy system? Or does refusal mean "you don't want to help yourself, so you need a longer stay in the hospital"? Who sets the policies for behaviors to be rewarded? What happens to patients if they refuse to participate? Are token economies used as a form of slave labor, along a sexist division of labor? Are token economy systems used only for women, as they were at the state hospital described by Levering?

Electroshock Therapy (EST)

Technically called *electroconvulsive therapy*, but more commonly known as *electroshock therapy*, EST is a "treatment" designed to eliminate depression by inducing convulsions in the patient. In EST therapy, the patient is supposed to be prepared with barbituates (as anesthesia) and muscle relaxants (to prevent fractures). Electricity is shot through the body of the patient through nodes attached to the temples. The voltage is not enough to kill a person, but it is enough to send the body into convulsions that resemble those of epileptics. EST, usually given in a series of treatments, is prescribed for people with severe depressions—they are supposed to "wake up" with the heavy mood lifted. "Treatments" often cause temporary disorientation and amnesia that can last at least two weeks (if not longer).[13]

EST was used a great deal in the fifties and not so much during the sixties. Now, however, it seems to be coming back into psychiatric fashion. Even though EST is frequently used as a quick form of therapy, researchers know little about how it works or what its long-term effects are. Why, for example, should convulsions have any effect on emotions? Even assuming that EST has a short-term effectiveness in lifting severe depression, does it keep depression from returning? It often causes temporary amnesia, but does it erase some memories permanently? Does it destroy any brain tissue or cause brain hemorrhaging? Why is it sometimes so painful? Do the number of treatments increase "effectiveness" or side effects? One puzzling thing that is known for sure is that EST causes tremendous *fear* in patients. People who have had treatments are often terrified of having them again—so much so that they will sometimes hide their problems so as to escape "therapy" by EST. Chesler quoted one woman's description:

> Also, I got scared of the shock treatments. It's a very scary feeling, especially when you feel like the metal things of the electricity goes through you—it's like a hammer hitting your head. I was afraid. . . .[14]

In her autobiographical novel *The Bell Jar*, Sylvia Plath described her first experience with EST:

> Doctor Gordon was fitting two metal plates on either side of my head. He buckled them into place with a strap that dented my forehead, and gave me a wire to bite.
>
> I shut my eyes.
>
> There was a brief silence, like an indrawn breath.
>
> Then something bent down and took hold of me and shook me like the end of the world. Whee-ee-ee-ee-ee, it shrilled, through an air crackling with blue light, and with each flash a great jolt drubbed me till I thought my bones would break and the sap fly out of me like a split plant.
>
> I wondered what terrible thing it was that I had done.[15]

Even in psychiatric circles, the controversy about EST—its effectiveness, its side-effects, its ethics—is not likely to be resolved soon.[16] But a more serious issue is how EST is being used in mental hospitals today. Like drugs, EST has become in some hospitals a substitute for other kinds of therapy—particularly therapy based on human contact and discussion of problems. With the contact between psychiatrists and patients at a minimum, many patients find that EST and drug "treatments" constitute the hospital's strategy for a "cure."

A woman who was committed to a mental hospital several times by her husband told Chesler:

> To make a long story short, this doctor didn't ask me my problem. All he did was give me a needle and put me to sleep. Then he kept giving me shock treatments ... this caused me to sleep all the time. Consequently, my children missed my attention and my husband enjoyed his freedom and had no guilt. This shock treatment went on for about six years. I was very subdued all the time and never objected to anything.[17]

Another woman told Chesler:

> The first thing [before the psychiatric interview] they did was give everyone shock treatment. It didn't matter who you were. You walked

in and they gave you shock three times a week. Before they decided what ward you were going in, they shocked you completely. I was scared to death. I thought I was going to die. . . . The only person who came to see me, and this is going to make you laugh a little bit, came to give me an I.Q. test.[18]

Within the context of individual mental institutions, there is considerable variation on a number of key issues that center on the *politics* of EST: Who decides whether EST should be given? Does a patient have the legal right to refuse EST? How often is it performed? Is it used more often on women? Old people? Poor people? Is it really given only to severely depressed patients? Are the muscle relaxants (necessary to prevent fractures) used in all cases? Certainly the potential for abuse of EST exists in mental hospitals. Since patients tend to fear it, EST can be a "treatment" used punitively to control unacceptable behavior.[19] One former patient even speculated that the economics of insurance benefits and hospital costs has indirectly contributed to the continuation of extensive ETS:

> In some private hospitals known as "shock shops," EST is almost the only form of "treatment" used. This is related to the fact that many insurance policies which cover psychiatric "care" cover only shock treatments. So the hospitals stand to collect a lot of money—the more "treatments," the more money.

Lobotomy and Other Kinds of Psychosurgery

A lobotomy is a form of psychosurgery used to destroy an area of the brain. *It is not reversible.* Its purpose is to eliminate the part of the brain that controls emotional behavior patterns that have been diagnosed as undesirable. The brain tissue is destroyed by techniques that constantly change or become more "sophisticated." Operations have been variously performed by incisions made through the temples, the eyes, by ultrasound, electrical coagulation, and implanted radium seeds. Today, other parts of the brain are removed instead of the lobes; technical names for some of these psychosurgeries are *amygdalotomies, thalèmotomies, diencephalotomies.*

During the thirties and forties, lobotomies were used mainly on state hospital patients with "chronic and disabling mental diseases." Some 50,000 Americans were lobotomized during this first wave. The operation was very crude and destroyed so much of the frontal lobe of the brain (the seat of emotion, creativity, and abstract thinking) that people became basically vegetables. During the fifties, lobotomies declined in popularity as the new electroshock therapy and drug therapy began to become popular.

But psychosurgery did *not* die out. In his article "The Return of Lobotomy and Psychosurgery" (a review of world literature on psychosurgery that he read into the Congressional Record in February, 1972), Dr. Peter Breggin, a psychiatrist who has been investigating psychosurgery, claims that we are in a second wave of psychosurgery popularity—lobotomies are on the rise for treating " 'overactive children,' depressed housewives, prisoners, homosexuals, addicts, alcoholics, and old people." Breggin writes that psychosurgeons themselves say that 400 to 600 operations are performed per year in the United States alone. Breggin asserts that psychosurgery is presently being advocated as a "treatment" to be used early in the "illness," *not* as a last resort. He notes that in one study, only 59 out of 300 people who were operated on were considered seriously ill.[20]

Who gets psychosurgery treatment now? Women, minority people, children, and prisoners are the new targets—and the diagnosis that sends them to the operating table is most often "neurotic" for women or "hyperactive" or "restless" for children. Lobotomized people can now leave the mental hospital, return to their homes, and lead "useful," quiet lives as nonrebellious housewives, factory workers, or obedient children.

Barbara Roberts wrote:

Dr. Freeman, the "dean of lobotomists," openly stated that lobotomized women make good housekeepers. . . . In Canada, Dr. Earle Baker of the University of Toronto reports the case of a promiscuous housewife who ran away from home frequently and sometimes became suicidal. After her lobotomy, her doctors bragged that she was *cured* of her promiscuity and was now a model housewife. Dr. Breggin contends that the reason women respond "better" to lobotomies is their passive conditioning, and adds that it is more socially acceptable to lobotomize women because creativity, which the operation totally destroys, is, to this society, an "expendable quality" in women. . . . Dr. Lindstrom, a prominent California neurosurgeon writing in 1964, said that 72 percent of psychotics and 80 percent of neurotics operated on are women. Seventy-one percent of the lobotomies performed by Drs. Brown and Lighthill in 1968 were on women. And Dr. R. F. Heatherton, at the Kingston Psychiatric Hospital in Ontario, admitted at a 1970 medical conference that the hospital administration refused to allow lobotomies on men because of the unfavorable publicity given to lobotomy in Canada; that publicity did not, however, deter the hospital from performing lobotomies on seventeen women. Repeatedly in the psychosurgical literature it is regarded as evidence of success if a previously distraught woman is able to return to housekeeping chores.[21]

What is the effect of the so-called greatly perfected and localized psychosurgery of the new wave? It is true that lobotomies often transform troublesome patients into models of good behavior—tranquil, calm, vacantly content; and that women with the "new" lobotomies can return home to care for their families—"model women." But even if psychosurgery will ever provide answers to "mental illness," the research today is still at a very crude stage. If you are lobotomized, you will be a guinea pig in the very early stages of psychosurgery for which understanding of the so-called "side effects" (which for you are the only effects that matter) is very limited. And even if these lobotomies today do leave a person with reasoning powers as the psychosurgeons claim, they still destroy unknown quantities of energy, vitality, sexual drive, spontaneity, decision-making ability, creativity, personality, and so forth *along* with the anger or depression the doctors want to eliminate.

Lobotomies are the most dangerous "treatment" you could confront in a mental hospital. No matter what scientific justifications the august psychosurgeons use to rationalize their actions, lobotomies have clearly been used for social, political, and punitive purposes.[22]

The people who make the decision to lobotomize people in mental institutions are likely to make this catastrophic recommendation on the basis of *their own* assumptions about what is "sane" behavior. They might not recognize your anger or depression about your life situation as justified. They may assume that a "sane" woman would cheerfully accept her duties in the home or work force.

One important question you should try to find the answer to in your state is this: What are your legal rights concerning psychosurgery? This varies by state; uninformed consent and outright bypassing of the patient appears to be common in many states. The same people who commit you, who control your daily life, or who keep you in the hospital may be the ones who literally hold the power of psychosurgery over your head.

CONDITIONS IN THE HOSPITAL

There is no uniform, standardized type of mental institution in this country. Conditions vary tremendously from institution to institution, as is true of clientele. If you foresee a stay in a mental hospital for yourself, you should do all you can to find out what the hospital is like, what it costs, who goes there, and what kinds of "treatment" programs it offers.

State and Private Hospitals

The main difference between public and private hospitals is cost. Private hospitals whose surroundings are sometimes very plush and where individual attention is somewhat more likely may cost as much as $30,000 a year. This doesn't even include fees for psychiatrists or occupational therapy. Few insurance policies cover such hospitalization. State hospitals, where conditions can be more brutal, often try to bill patients (about $130 a week). Public institutions tend to release patients faster. They also tend to use less electroshock therapy.

Questions about conditions in state versus private institutions include the following: What is the average difference in staff-to-patient ratios? How much money is normally spent per patient? Which place is more likely to try innovative techniques? Or potentially harmful techniques? Which place is more custodial? How long do women normally stay in each kind of institution?

Kinds of People in Mental Hospitals

The proportion of poor, Black, and other minority women to white, middle-class women in mental institutions is much greater than their proportions in society at large. It's probable that many of the poor women who wind up in mental hospitals would be seeing a therapist once a week instead, as middle-class women do, if they had more money. Questions relating to the kinds of people in mental institutions directly relate to the money factor: Are third-world women, for example, likely to stay in an institution *longer* than middle-class women? Is their care more custodial? How does the triple oppression— race, sex, and class—affect the type of treatment they get? How do the hospital's notions of the proper goals for women contrast with the realities of their life—are they being trained to be submissive and dependent even when they are the main support of the family? Are they encouraged to change their appearance when their only job "opportunity" may be menial jobs?

Labor in the Mental Hospitals

Many ex-patients assert that mental hospitals couldn't function without the labor (which often goes by the name "industrial therapy") of mental patients. Pay for such labor varies from state to state, but is generally very low and sometimes even nonexistent. Patients often do the work out of sheer boredom. One of the damaging effects jobs that help run the hospital can have is to condition a person to accept similar work outside the hospital. Staff members are likely to think that you are only suitable for that kind of work. One ex-patient told us:

> *At the hospital, I was told that if I would wear a skirt I could get a job in the hospital typing for a psychology research project. I was doing good work for the doctor/professor and I quietly hoped that he might help me somehow. He was impressed with my work and with the fact that I had been to college. One day when we got to talking, his advice to me was—"You'd make a wonderful secretary. Why don't you look for a good secretarial job when you get well?"*

Most work in the hospital is not nearly as interesting as working for a researcher; it is mostly domestic work assigned along stereotypical sex-role lines.

> I was proud to be the private housekeeper for Dr. X. I cleaned and cooked, baby-sat, shopped and even tutored her son in Spanish. . . . What I didn't like was having to wash their underwear. That I didn't like. . . . I used to go out to work just to get out . . . you mop floors, you make beds, you wash windows, you wash floors . . . the only place they pay you is the commissary. Ten dollars a month for food. I worked there also. . . . Also, a lot of other places were worse. They had a laundry there, and let me tell you, you work hard there.[23]

Conditions may vary from institution to institution, but it is important to know what forms of job training, if any, are offered in mental institutions. Is any of the forced labor useful to people once they leave the hospital? What happens to you if you refuse to do the forced labor?

> I refused to peel potatoes in the kitchen. So they threw me in solitary for a few days.[24]

And what happens to women who excel at their labor in the hospital? Are they ever kept from release because they work so well the staff doesn't want to lose them?

MENTAL HOSPITALS: SHOULD YOU EVER GO?

The picture we have painted of mental hospitals is grim, for the dangers can be great. But like therapy on the outside, mental hospitals vary enormously in their potential for serious harm or even good—much depends on the individual institutions and staff and on the strengths of the patient. But being in a mental hospital *can* leave scars and insecurities that may take years to overcome. Some women feel that their institutionalization *created* problems worse than their original ones.

If you are considering admitting yourself to a hospital, only you can judge whether you are desperate enough to risk the hospital experience. Your own suffering, fear, or isolation may outweigh the problems emerging from being tagged with the label "crazy." In making your decision, however, don't look at a mental hospital as a peaceful sanitarium where kind experts will swarm about you, eager to help. No matter how good or "progressive" a hospital might be, it will have its own pressures and difficulties, many of which will require all your strength to deal with. If you face commitment by parents, husband, or relatives, you simply have no choice.

The purpose of this chapter has not been to make recommendations about whether you should go to a mental institution. It has been rather to warn you of the difficulties you might face if you do go or find yourself committed to a hospital. Perhaps the best way to end this section on mental institutions is first with the account of a woman who was both badly scarred and later helped in a mental hospital and then with a letter written to us concerning this account.

I had been in various mental institutions for several years and found them totally dehumanizing and destructive. They only increased my withdrawal, self-hate, and self-blame until one day a woman therapist asked me if I would accept therapy with her. It was a special thing to be chosen by a therapist in this way, especially since so few patients had any opportunity to talk regularly with a therapist one-to-one. This psychiatrist was always warm and supportive. She helped to create in me a growing belief that maybe I wasn't as bad, valueless, or without identity as I had felt. My therapist showed respect for me, often praising me for my sensitivity—"You just had a good insight. I didn't think of that." A mutual respect and caring was a part of our talk, because the therapist was not afraid to admit that her "patient" was teaching her things too. She even said that if she faced a crisis in her life, she would think of going into therapy with her "patient."

It's honest to include this experience [in your book], but I think ending the chapter on an up note is too optimistic. Good things like that last story do happen, but very *rarely. Most women are devastated by the hospital experience. People often ask me if I got anything at all out of my experience in the hospital (psychology students most often ask this question) as if they can't believe that those giant institutions, built by taxpayers' money, and supposedly places of humane care and treatment, are in reality places of torture. The best thing I got out of being committed to a hospital was an indelible knowledge of the lengths to which this society will go to punish people who don't conform, and a good understanding of how power in a patriarchy is exercised. I understand how psychiatry, in the guise of benevolence, systematically dehumanizes people in hospitals, until they are nothing but broken souls, shells who walk and utter words but who have been stripped of all emotional life and all sense of self. They are patched together well enough to go out and work, or perform the duties of wives and mothers—institutional psychiatry in the arena of the hospital is the soft police force of the ruling class.*

Another thing I saw in the hospital were the patients from the chronic wards, people who'd been there 30 or 40 years—and the cemetary on the hospital grounds, where there were no names on the tombstones, only the number from the hospital record. I can have no more illusions about what can happen to you if you don't make it in this society in one way or another. My hospital experience provides my basic frame of reference in my attempts to survive from day to day.

FOOTNOTES

¹See Phyllis Chesler, *Women and Madness* (New York: Doubleday, 1972), pp. 35, 169, 160–80; Thomas S. Szasz, *Ideology and Insanity: Essays on the Psychiatric Dehumanization of Man* (New York: Doubleday, 1970), pp. 113–39; Erving Goffman, "The Medical Model and Mental Hospitalization," in Phil Brown, ed. *Radical Psychology* (New York: Harper & Row, 1973), pp. 38–39; David Rosenhan, "On Being Sane in Insane Places," *Science*, 179 (January 19, 1973), 250–58; and a summary of Rosenhan's study by Jackie Cristeve, "The Rosenhan Experiment: Psychiatric Myths Exposed," *Rough Times*, 3, no. 4 (February–March 1973), p. 8.

²Chesler, pp. 163–80. For a description of how "acting out" is punished, see Anonymous, "Ordeal in a Mental Hospital," in *Rough Times*, produced by Jerome Agel (New York: Ballantine Books, 1973), pp. 8–21. For a discussion of beating and brutality in mental institutions, see also Rosenhan, "On Being Sane in Insane Places," pp. 255–56.

³Rosenhan, "On Being Sane in Insane Places," p. 251. All following quotations from Rosenhan's study come from the same article.

⁴See especially Thomas Szasz, *Ideology and Insanity: Essays on the Psychiatric Dehumanization of Man*, pp. 12–24, 113–39; Good Times/Liberation News Service, "Vacaville: Lobotomies, Shock Therapy, and Torture for 'Violent' California Prisoners," in *Rough Times*, pp.206–208.

⁵Phyllis Chesler, *Women and Madness* (New York: Doubleday, 1972), pp. 166–75. Excerpts from *Women and Madness* by Phyllis Chesler. Copyright © 1972 by Phyllis Chesler. Reprinted by permission of Doubleday & Company, Inc. and Penguin Books Ltd.

⁶Susan Dworkin Levering, "She Must Be Some Kind of Nut," *Rough Times*, 3, no. 1 (September 1972), 3.

⁷Pauline Bart, "Depression in Middle-Aged Women," in *Women in Sexist Society*, Vivian Gornick and Barbara K. Moran, eds. (New York: Basic Books, 1971).

⁸See "The Theft of Life" in *Akwesasne Notes* (September 1977), p. 30 and "Killing Our Future: Sterilization & Experiments" in *Akwesasne Notes* (Spring 1977), pp. 4–6. Statistics for Native American women are based on a U.S. General Accounting Office study (1977). Write *Akwesasne Notes*, Mohawk Nation, via-Rooseveltown, N.Y. 13683, for copies. See also Irene Brody and Jennifer Lewis, "The Rising Abuse of Sterilization," *Guardian* (January 4, 1978), p. 8.

⁹Phil Brown, "Social Change at Harrowdale State Hospital: Impression II," in *Rough Times*, p. 37.

¹⁰Robert Seidenberg, M.D., 1971, in Chesler, *Women and Madness*, p. 167. For a discussion of drugs in mental hospitals, see also Rosenhan, "On Being Sane in Insane Places," p. 256; Judy Greenberg, "Become Mentally Healthy or I'll Kill You," in *Rough Times*, pp. 53–56; Phil Brown, "Social Change at Harrowdale State Hospital: Impression II," p. 36.

¹¹See also "Aversion Therapy: Straight at Any Price," *Rough Times*, 3, no. 4 (February–March 1973), 18.

¹²Levering, "She Must Be Some Kind of Nut," p. 3.

¹³Lothar Kalinowsky, "The Convulsive Therapies," in *Comprehensive Textbook of Psychiatry*, Alfred M. Freedman and Harold I. Kaplan, eds. (Baltimore, Md.: William & Wilkins, 1967), pp. 1279–85.

¹⁴Chesler, *Women and Madness*, p. 225.

[15]Sylvia Plath, *The Bell Jar* (New York: Bantam Books, 1971), pp. 119-20. Her first EST, done around 1953, seems to have been done without anesthesia or muscle relaxants. The later series of EST treatments she received were painless; but they still left her afraid, pp. 175-76.

[16]See Carl Salzman, "Electroconvulsive Therapy," in *Harvard Guide to Modern Psychiatry*, Armand M. Nicholi, Jr., ed. (Cambridge, Mass.: Harvard University Press, 1978), pp. 471-79.

[17]Chesler, *Women and Madness*, p. 166.

[18]Ibid, p. 167.

[19]See Anonymous, "Ordeal in a Mental Hospital," pp. 17-18; Greenberg, "Become Mentally Healthy or I'll Kill You," p. 56; Christopher Z. Hobson, "Surviving Psychotherapy," in *Rough Times*, p. 172; Good Times/Liberation News Service, "Vacaville: Lobotomies, Shock Therapy, and Torture for 'Violent' California Prisoners." p. 206.

[20]Breggin's argument is summarized in Barbara Roberts, "Psychosurgery: The Final Solution to the Woman Problem," *Rough Times*, 3, no. 1 (September 1972), 16-17. The reference for Breggin's report is: Dr. Peter Breggin, "The Return of Lobotomy and Psychosurgery," 188 Cong. Rec. Ext. of Remarks, Sect. 1602 (1972). See also Liberation News Service, "Lobotomies Are Back," in *Rough Times*, pp. 198-203.

[21]Ibid, p. 16.

[22]See ibid.; Thomas S. Szasz, *Ideology and Insanity*, pp. 12-24, 69-79, 113-40; see Chicago People's Law Office, "Check Out Your Mind," *Rough Times*, 3, no. 5 (April-May 1973), pp. 2-3, 17, 20 for a discussion of how psychosurgery is used in prisons as well as mental hospitals; Good Times/Liberations New Service, "Vacaville: Lobotomies, Shock Therapy, and Torture for 'Violent' California Prisoners," pp. 206-208.

[23]Chesler, *Women and Madness*, pp. 168, 226-27.

[24]Ibid., p. 168.

Resources

FEMINIST REFERRAL SERVICES*

Some cities have feminist referral services which provide a list of therapists that members of the service groups think will be good for women. If you cannot find a referral service where you live, you might try finding a woman's center or calling a local NOW (National Organization for Women) chapter. These groups might have a list of good therapists or might even offer informal or formal therapy by lay or professional women. Here are just a few such feminist referral services and therapy collectives—we are sure there are more:

NATIONAL

Feminist Therapy Roster, Nechama Liss-Levinson (National co-ordinator) Department of Psychiatry, Room 2313 Lab Office Building, SUNY, Stony Brook, NY 11794. The Roster divides the country into areas, each

*Addresses accurate as of 1977.

with a coordinator who screens those requesting to be listed and who updates the files. For referrals in your area, contact your area coordinator. Names and addresses are in the KNOW publication of the Association of Women in Psychology Feminist Therapy Roster (available for 10¢ from KNOW, P.O. Box 86031, Pittsburgh, PA 15221).

The People's Yellow Pages Published by Vocations for Social Change, 353 Broadway, Cambridge, MA 02139. Can be purchased in most bookstores.

The *New Woman's Survival Sourcebook*, Kristen Grimstad and Susan Rennie, eds., has a section on feminist referral and therapy groups. Available in most book stores.

NEW YORK

The Consultation Center for Women, 228 East 68th Street, New York, NY 10021 Telephone: (212) 724-7400

Women's Counseling Project at Columbia, Room 112, Earl Hall, Columbia University, 117th Street and Broadway, New York, NY 10027 Telephone: (212) 280-5113

Women's Institute for Psychotherapy, 105 West 13th Street, New York, NY 10011 Telephone: (212) 741-1278

The Feminist Collective, Box 442, Planetarium Station, New York, NY 10024

The Feminist Center for Human Growth and Development, Inc., Suite 1-C, 40 East 68th Street, New York, NY 10021 Telephone: (212) 535-8505

MASSACHUSETTS

Women's Counseling and Resource Center, 1555 Massachusetts Avenue, Cambridge, MA 02138 Telephone: (617) 492-8568

Womanspace: Feminist Therapy Collective, Inc., 636 Beacon Street, Boston, MA 02115 They publish "New England Directory of Women Counselors and Psychotherapists"; "Counseling Women: A Bibliography" (1975); "Issues in the Counseling and Psychology of Women" (1976); and "Women: Sexuality, Psychology and Psychotherapy."

Women and Therapy Collective of the Goddard–Cambridge Graduate Program in Social Change 1974–1975. Publishes "Off the Couch: A Woman's Guide to Therapy." This may be ordered from *State and Mind*, Box 89, West Somerville, MA 02144. Send $2 plus 25¢ for handling.

MICHIGAN

Women's Crisis Center, 325 East Summit Street, Ann Arbor, MI 48104 Telephone: (313) 994-9100 (crisis), 761-9475 (business)

Tapestry 802 Monroe, Ann Arbor, MI 48104

OHIO

The Women's Growth Co-Operative, P.O. Box 18472, Cleveland Heights, OH 44118 Telephone: (216) 321-8582

Cleveland Women's Counseling, P.O. Box 18472, Cleveland, OH 44118 Telephone: (216) 321-8585

MINNESOTA

Chrysalis Women's Center, 2104 Stevens Avenue, South Minneapolis, MN 55404 Telephone: (612) 871-0118

Sagaris, 2619 Garfield Avenue, South Minneapolis, MN 55408 Telephone: (612) 825-7338

PENNSYLVANIA

Feminist Therapy Collective, 2132 Lombard Street, Philadelphia, PA 19146 Telephone: (215) 546-1234

CONNECTICUT

Women's Therapy Referral Service, 42 Main Street, Southport, CT 06490 Telephone: (203) 255-5350

ILLINOIS

Chicago chapter, Association for Women in Psychology, Publishers of "Psychological Karate: How to Deal with Sexism in Groups" and "How to Tell if Your Therapist's Sexism is Interfering With Your Treatment." These pamphlets may be ordered for 30¢ each plus a self-addressed stamped envelope from Behavioral Research Fund, 1140 South Paulina Street, Chicago, IL 60612, Attn: Anne M. Seiden, M.D.

MENTAL PATIENTS' ORGANIZATIONS AND RESOURCES

KIN 77

Write to Nancy Hess, 7025 Woolston Road, Philadelphia, PA 19138.

A resource guide for the "emotionally restored mentally ill" woman and a section for those elderly women in the Philadelphia area. Hard-cover is $4.50 and soft is $2.50.

NETWORK AGAINST PSYCHIATRIC ASSAULT

Publish *The History of Shock Treatment* and *Madness Network News*. 2150 Market Street, San Francisco, CA 94114.

PATIENT ADVOCACY LEGAL SERVICE (PALS)

Washington University Law School, St. Louis, MO 63130. They operate a clearinghouse for information in the mental commitment area.

PATIENTS' RIGHTS ORGANIZATION

2108 Payne Avenue, Room 707, Cleveland, OH 44114. (216) 795-7825 evenings. This is an action group open to current, former or potential victims of emotional or nervous illness. Its purpose is to advocate better living conditions for patients and housing for ex-patients, to investigate job discrimination against ex-patients, to promote general rights of patients and ex-patients, and to provide community education regarding public attitude toward the plight of emotional illness victims. Group published a newsletter— *Nervous Breakthrough*. Subscription is $2 donation. Group also publishes *Guidelines for Psychotherapeutic Drugs* and *Mental Patients' Handbook of Legal Rights*.

PROJECT RELEASE

202 Riverside Drive, Apt. 4E, New York, NY 10025. A supportive community of former psychiatric inmates. Publish "Consumer's Guide to Psychiatric Medication" and a newsletter *We Are Silent No Longer*. Newsletter donation is $2.

PROJECT RENAISSANCE

8614 Euclid Avenue (basement of Emmanual Episcopal Church), Cleveland, OH 44016. (216) 229-5200. An outgrowth of Patients' Rights Organization, this is a self-help mental cooperative. All volunteers are former mental patients. Main services are information and referral. Classes and social events.

WELCOME BACK

3206 Prospect Avenue, Cleveland, OH 44115. Newsletter and information exchange for people who have had mental hospital experiences. Subscription is $5 donation, free with a letter about your life, experiences, problems. Letters forwarded (enclose 25¢).

There are many more groups than those listed. Because only organizations we were certain were in existence are included, we suggest you write to *Madness Network News*, *State and Mind*, or *Issues in Radical Therapy* (all listed in bibliography) for information about groups in your area.

ANNOTATED BIBLIOGRAPHY

We can come to understand our past and work to shape a new future by talking openly with other women. Often this sharing itself creates an exhilarating sense of liberation just because hidden feelings and ideas have "come out of the closet" and found sympathetic listeners. But we can also expand the horizons of change by reading. What follows is an annotated list of books that might be useful to you. It is *not* meant to be an exhaustive list, nor does it imply a negative judgment of the many important books that are not included. It is meant to provide a starting point for your reading.

Psychology of Women:
Feminist and Nonfeminist Sources

Bem, Sandra L. and Daryl J. Bem, "Training the Woman to Know Her Place: The Power of the Non-Conscious Ideology," In Michelle Hoffnung Garskof's *Roles Women Play: Readings Toward Women's Liberation*. Belmont, Cal.: Brooks/Cole, 1971. Paperback. This is one of the very best and most easily readable articles on the power of socialization. The Bems' thesis is that the dominant norms of any given culture are internalized by people so subtly and gradually that they operate as a "nonconscious ideology," telling us what is "natural" and "appropriate" for men and women to do. This article was crucial to our developing sense that therapists (just like all of us) have very deep-seated, often unconscious presuppositions about women that are bound to enter into therapy no matter how "liberated" they are.

Brodsky, Annette and Jean Holroyd, et. al, "Report of the Task Force on Sex Bias and Sex-Role Stereotyping in Psychotherapeutic Practice," April 1975. This report was authorized by the Board of Professional Affairs (BPA) of the American Psychological Association (APA). It examines the extent and manner of sex bias and sex-role stereotyping in psychotherapeutic practice and recommends actions for the APA and therapists to take to reduce sex bias in therapy. It contains a good bibliography. Order copies from the American Psychological Association, 1200 17th St. N.W., Washington, D.C. 20036.

Broverman, Inge K. and Donald Broverman, et al., "Sex-Role Stereotypes and Clinical Judgments of Mental Health," *Journal of Consulting and Clinical Psychology*, 34, no. 1 (1970), 1-7. The Broverman study is based on a sex-role stereotype questionnaire given to therapists. The response indicated that personality traits considered "masculine" were traits associated with psychologically "normal" adults, while traits considered "feminine" were associated with psychologically unhealthy adults. The study showed how extensively many therapists have either consciously or unconsciously accepted traditional definitions of "masculine" and "feminine."

Brown, Phil, ed., *Radical Psychology*. New York: Harper, 1973. Paperback. This interesting anthology includes basic articles by Franz Fanon (psychology of oppression), Karl Marx (alienation), Wilhelm Reich (sexual struggle and repression), R. D. Laing, Thomas Szasz (myths of mental illness), Naomi Weisstein (social science constructs female identity), Radicalesbians ("woman-identified woman"), etc. In addition, the book has a section of personal accounts of experiences in therapy and a section on the efforts of radical therapists and clients to change the system.

Chesler, Phyllis, "Men Drive Woman Crazy," *Psychology Today*, 5, no. 2 (July 1971). Chesler discusses the reasons women go into therapy, compares men and women in therapy and their preferences for male or female therapists, and shows, as does the Broverman study, what therapists think are "proper" roles for women and men.

Chesler, Phyllis, *Women and Madness*. New York: Doubleday, 1972. Hardback and paperback. This book, often painful to read, is an indictment of the institution of therapy. It contains much information, including statistics, about women in mental institutions (commitment, conditions, etc.), poor and third-world women. Chesler uses graphs, charts, studies, personal accounts, interviews, and the mother-daughter myth of Demeter and Persephone to illustrate her material.

Chorover, Stephan L., "The Pacification of the Brain," *Psychology Today*, 7, no. 12 (May 1974), 59-69. This article contains much technical information on lobotomy and argues that this technique does not even "succeed" within the inhumanly limited definition of "success" used by psychosurgeons. Chorover contends lobotomized people become totally disoriented, confused, unable to solve simple problems, often having hallucinations—in short the operation destroys their ability to "function" in society.

Cox, Sue, *Female Psychology: The Emerging Self*. Chicago: Science Research Associates, 1976. Paperback. This is a good anthology of articles on the psychology of women. It includes sections on sex differences, socialization (see especially Bem and Bem's "Case Study of a Nonconscious Ideology"), minority women, sexuality. One section on psychotherapy and women analyzes the assumption of many therapists that the traditional wife-mother role makes women happy. The book has many interesting illustrations and brief quotations. (See especially psychologist Annette Brodsky's article, "The Consciousness-Raising Group as a Model for Therapy With Women.")

Deutsch, Hélène, *The Psychology of Women: A Psychoanalytic Interpretation*, Vols. I and II. New York: Grune & Stratton, 1944. Hardback and paperback. Deutsch, a longtime associate of Freud, published this statement of female psychosexual development and personality after Freud's death. But it is an extension and expansion of Freud's basic theories on girls and women.

Franks, Violet and Burtle Vasanti, eds., *Women in Therapy: New Psychotherapies for a Changing Society*. New York: Brunner/Mazel, 1974. This anthology of essays written by psychologists and sociologists is primarily directed to a professional audience, but it provides a scholarly coverage of many of the issues discussed in this book. It includes sections on the history of therapeutic approaches to women; biological and cultural influences on sex roles; therapy with depressed, phobic, and alcoholic women; contemporary schools of therapy (e.g., behavior therapy, gestalt therapy, etc.); and women and mental institutions.

Freud, Sigmund, *An Outline of Psychoanalysis*, tran. James Strachey. 1939; rpt. New York: Norton, 1949. Paperback. See Chapter Seven, "An Example of Psychoanalytic Work," pp. 80-99, for Freud's summation of his theory of women.

Freud, Sigmund, *New Introductory Lectures on Psychoanalysis*, tran. James Strachey. 1933; rpt. New York: Norton, 1964. Paperback. See especially "Femininity," pp. 112–135. This lecture was based on two earlier papers: "Some Psychical Consequences of the Anatomical Distinction Between the Sexes" (1925) and "Female Sexuality" (1931), both of which can be found in his collected works.

Garskof, Michelle Hoffnung, ed., *Roles Women Play: Readings Toward Women's Liberation*. Belmont, Cal.: Brooks/Cole, 1971. Paperback. This collection contains many of the best-known articles on women, including Naomi Weisstein's "Psychology Constructs the Female," Sandra Bem's and Daryl Bem's "Training the Women to Know Her Place: The Power of the Non-Conscious Ideology," Alice Rossi's "Equality Between the Sexes: An Immodest Proposal," Margaret Benston's "The Political Economy of Women's Liberation." Garskof arranged this collection for courses on the psychology of women, as well as for general reading; she has "stressed the interrelationship of economic and social factors in the evolution of the psychology of women."

Halleck, Seymour L., *The Politics of Therapy*. New York: Science House, 1971. Written by a psychiatrist on a university campus during the most intense years of student rebellion, this book offers some introduction to the politics of psychotherapy (including individual and group therapy, family therapy, drug therapy, behavior therapy, etc.). It contains very little on women and therapy, because Halleck writes in terms of the male client. He describes his position as a "middle" ground between conservative and radical therapy.

Harding, M. Esther, *Woman's Mysteries: Ancient and Modern: A Psychological Interpretation of the Feminine Principle as Portrayed in Myth, Story and Dreams*. New York: Bantam, 1971. Paperback. This book, often placed in the "women's sections" of bookstores, is written entirely from the Jungian, analytical psychological perspective. It illustrates the belief that woman's biology determines her "feminine" nature and role. (Woman's desire for emancipation, Harding believes, will destroy her "innate" capacity for subjectivity and human relatedness.)

Horner, Matina S., "Femininity and Successful Achievement: A Basic Inconsistency," in Michelle Hoffnung Garskof's *Roles Women Play: Readings Toward Women's Liberation*. Belmont, Cal.: Brooks/Cole, 1971. Paperback. This important article argues that women are often more afraid of succeeding than they are of failing because achievement (especially in traditionally male areas) is not considered "feminine." Her thesis has very wide-reaching implications for the psychology of women and for successful therapy.

Horney, Karen, *Feminine Psychology*, ed. Harold Kelman. New York: Norton, 1967. Paperback. This collection of some of Horney's most important essays on the psychology of women simultaneously demonstrates her ties to psychoanalytic theory and her attack on Freud's theories about women. She forcefully argued in Freud's own "territory" that whatever deficiencies, inadequacies, or masochism women might feel originate in socialization and the societal situation of women, not in biology.

Jongeward, Dorothy and Dru Scott. *Women as Winners: Transactional Analysis for Personal Growth.* Reading, Mass./Menlo Park, Cal.: Addison-Wesley, 1976. Paperback. Written for a general audience of women who are interested in personal growth, this book represents a mix of the theories and techniques of transactional analysis and gestalt therapy. Each section contains the authors' description of problem areas in women's growth; examples of actual women and recommendation of what women with each problem should do to change; and a "Steps to Awareness" checklist of questions women can ask about themselves. However, the authors perpetuate the idea that the only thing between a woman and emancipation is her own inability to change.

Kaplan, Alexandra G. and Joan P. Bean, eds., *Beyond Sex-Role Stereotypes: Readings Toward a Psychology of Androgyny.* Boston: Little, Brown & Co., 1976. Paperback. This book on the psychology of women is often quite technical, but if you are interested in what the women's studies psychologists are saying about the distorted psychologies of the past and the potentially liberating psychologies being developed now, this is a useful book. See especially Alexandra Kaplan's article, "Androgyny as a Model of Mental Health for Women: From Theory to Therapy," which discusses the application of feminist theory to therapy.

Mander, Anica Vessel and Anne Kent Rush, *Feminism as Therapy.* New York: Random House, 1974. Paperback. Written by a feminist and a feminist body therapist, the book describes the potential of feminism to heal the suffering caused by a male-dominated society. Feminism is seen as a kind of therapy that teaches women to see the political context of their personal lives. The book contains some useful exercises, particularly in body work.

Osborn, Susan M. and Gloria Harris, *Assertive Training for Women.* Springfield, Ill.: Thomas, 1975. Paperback. This book about assertiveness training for women places this behavior therapy squarely within the context of feminism. The authors' description of the techniques of assertive training (exercises, homework, role-playing, etc.) begins with their analysis of why women particularly need such training. Although the book is not meant to be a guide to show women how to develop assertiveness by themselves, it is a comprehensive introduction to the analyses and techniques of feminist assertiveness training.

Phelps, Stanlee and Nancy Austin, *The Assertive Woman.* San Luis Obispo, Cal., 1975. Paperback. This book is a guidebook on assertiveness training, written informally and directly so that women can try some of the techniques without joining an assertiveness training group. It contains discussions and analysis of such topics as assertive behaviors, assertive body image, assertive attitudes, saying "no," asserting sensuality, etc.

Piercy, Marge, *Woman on the Edge of Time.* New York: Knopf, 1976. Paperback. This is a compelling novel about a Chicana who is labeled insane and committed to a state mental hospital. Through her, readers share the horrors of a mental institution and the joys of a possible androgynous society in which men and women are encouraged to realize their full potential, one not dependent on their sex.

The Radical Therapist Collective, produced by Jerome Agel. *The Radical Therapist.* New York: Ballantine, 1971. Paperback. This book is an anthology of essays drawn from the early issues of the journal, *The Radical Therapist.* It includes articles on therapy as an institution, radical therapy, consciousness-raising, women's groups, female sexuality, lesbianism, and various manifestos. According to this anthology, the analysis of existing therapy and the basis for a new therapy can be summarized thus: therapy *has* meant "adjustment"; therapy *should* mean "political change."

Rawlings, Edna I. and Dianne K. Carter, eds., *Psychotherapy for Women: Treatment Toward Equality* (Springfield, Ill.: Charles C. Thomas, 1977). This is the best all-around scholarly book on psychotherapy for women. It includes articles on the following topics: feminist and nonsexist psychotherapy; nonsexist approaches to psychotherapy for women; assertion training for women; career counseling; psychotherapy for lesbians; feminism as therapy; radical feminism as a challenge to professional psychotherapy; and social activism as therapy.

The Rough Times Staff, produced by Jerome Agel, *Rough Times* (New York: Ballantine Books, 1973). Paperback. This volume is the second anthology . . . produced of . . . writings taken from the journal *Rough Times* (formerly *The Radical Therapist*). It includes articles on mental hospitals, professionalism, and mental health as oppression.

Szasz, Thomas S., *Ideology and Insanity: Essays on the Psychiatric Dehumanization of Man.* New York: Anchor, 1970. Paperback. This collection presents a strong statement of psychiatrist Szasz's basic position: that therapy is not a "science"; as a replacement of religion, its definitions of "mental illness" constitute an ideology of "normal," "healthy" behavior that rationalizes the needs of the system to keep people in line. Therapy as an institution serves the state and inhibits human freedom.

Tennov, Dorothy, *Psychotherapy: The Hazardous Cure.* New York: Anchor, 1975. Paperback. This is an important book by a feminist psychologist which contains a wide-ranging and knowledgeable discussion of the institution of psychotherapy. It includes sections on Freud, varieties of therapies (including feminist therapy), women and psychotherapy, how the profession operates (training, licensing, fees, etc.), relationship of psychotherapy to research, psychotherapy as social control, and so forth.

Williams, Elizabeth Friar, *Notes of a Feminist Therapist*. New York: Praeger, 1976. Hardback. This is an exceptional book about feminist therapy. With many descriptions of actual women in therapy, it will give readers a good sense of what is involved in nontraditional feminist therapy. It explores subjects such as women and love, sex, motherhood, loneliness, depression, roles women play, creativity, and anger.

General Books and Anthologies

Boston Women's Health Collective, *Our Bodies, Ourselves, A Book By and For Women*, 2nd ed. New York: Simon & Schuster, 1976. Paperback. Although this superb book has little specific material on therapy or "mental" health, it has long, useful sections filled with factual information and personal accounts on relationships, sexuality, lesbian experience, birth control, abortion, pregnancy, lactation, nutrition, menopause, rape, veneral disease, etc. Besides providing a wealth of essential physiological information about our bodies, the book also offers an understanding of how important women's *feelings* are.

Daly, Mary, *The Church and the Second Sex*. New York: Harper, 1968. Paperback. In this book Daly attacks the sexism of the church, seeing religion as a source of socialization into traditional values about women's nature, sexuality, and roles. (See also Daly's book, *Beyond God the Father: Toward a Philosophy of Feminism* [1973].)

de Beauvoir, Simone, *The Second Sex*. 1949; rpt. New York: Bantam, 1961. Paperback. Perhaps no book on feminist theory is as comprehensive as this philosophical exploration of the causes and conditions of women's subordinate position. The book includes discussions of the impact of biological sex differences, women in history, women in literature, and contemporary women's lives throughout the life cycle. (See especially her critique of Freud and psychoanalysis, pp. 33–46.)

Firestone, Shulamith, *The Dialectic of Sex: The Case for Feminist Revolution*. New York: Bantam, 1970. Paperback. In addition to Firestone's critique of Freud (pp. 41–72), this book provides an important theoretical statement about the causes and conditions of the suppression of women. Firestone argues that biology—woman's reproductive nature —is the cause of her domination; now technology, properly used, can free women from unwanted pregnancy. Her discussion of the mystique of romantic love is valuable.

Freeman, Jo, *Women: A Feminist Perspective*. Palo Alto, Cal.: Mayfield, 1975. Paperback. This collection of essays is one of the best and most comprehensive anthologies in women's studies. It includes articles on women's bodies, the family, socialization, women's work, images of women, institutions of social control, and feminism. Susan Griffin's "Rape: The All-American Crime" is one of the best short essays on rape available; see also Phyllis Chesler's "Marriage and Psychotherapy," Pauli Murray's "The Liberation of Black Women," and Pauline Bart's "The Loneliness of the Long-Distance Runner."

Friedan, Betty, *The Feminine Mystique*. New York: Norton, 1963. Paper-
    back. This book, which led to the founding in 1966 of NOW, explores
    the psychological stresses and contradictions in the lives of mainly
    middle-class, educated women. "The Problem That Has No Name"
    is an especially eloquent statement of the emptiness many educated
    women face as their lives are defined by their wife–mother role. The
    chapter on Freud and functionalism is a fine critique.

Gornick, Vivian and Barbara K. Moran, eds., *Women in Sexist Society,
    Studies in Power and Powerlessness*. New York: Basic Books, 1971.
    Paperback. This is an excellent collection of informative essays. (See
    especially Pauline Bart's, "Depression in Middle-Aged Women,"
    based on painful interviews with women in mental institutions; Jessie
    Bernard's, "The Paradox of the Happy Marriage"; Phyllis Chesler's,
    "Patient and Patriarch: Women in the Psychotherapeutic relation-
    ship"; Alix Shulman's, "Organs and Orgasms"; and Naomi Weisstein's,
    "Psychology Constructs the Female.")

Greer, Germaine, *The Female Eunuch*. New York: Bantam Books, 1970.
    Paperback. Greer's exploration of the sexual and sex-role dimensions
    of women's oppression includes a discussion of "Body" or female
    sexuality; "Soul," or the creation of the myth of the Eternal Feminine;
    "Love," or the ideology of romantic love; "Hate," or the abuse and
    mutilation of women; and "Revolution"—Greer's proposals for change.
    The book is well-known for its argument that a male-dominated
    society has repressed a genuine female sexuality as a way of keeping
    women "in their place." Greer argues that women are socialized into
    being "eunuchs," impotent in both private and public spheres. Her
    chapter "The Psychological Sell" is useful for an analysis of the role
    of psychology in perpetuating traditional concepts of "the feminine."

Koedt, Anne, Ellen Levine, and Anita Rapone, eds., *Radical Feminism*.
    New York: Quadrangle, 1973. Paperback. This is an extremely useful
    collection with some forty articles that have emerged out of the con-
    temporary feminist movement. It includes sections on women's ex-
    perience, theory and analysis, building a movement, and the arts.
    Pamela Allen's article on consciousness-raising groups, "Free Space,"
    is a good introduction to "CR."

Martin, Del, *Battered Wives*. San Francisco, Cal.: Glide, 1976. Paperback.
    This book provides a general introduction to and analysis of wife-
    beating, and by extension, physical aggression against women in gen-
    eral. It includes some historical material on marriage contracts, the
    psychology of the batterer and the woman who stays with him, prob-
    lems with the legal system and social services, survival tactics and
    refuges for battered women.

Millett, Kate, *Sexual Politics*. New York: Avon, 1969. Paperback. This
    important book in feminist theory presents Millett's explanation of
    sexual politics—the power relations between men and women—and
    historical analysis (1830–1960) of the origins of the sexual revolution

and counterrevolution. Her critique of Freud, post-Freudians, and functionalism (pp. 176–235) is particularly useful.

Morgan, Robin, ed., *Sisterhood Is Powerful: An Anthology of Writings from the Women's Liberation Movement.* New York: Vintage, 1970. Paperback. This was one of the first anthologies to come out of the women's movement, and it is still one of the best all-round introductions to feminist issues. It includes articles on women in the professions; the psychological and sexual repression of women; the experiences of black and Chicana women; women in high schools; women and aging; women and the media; and so forth. The final sections include poems, manifestos, and articles outlining aspects of social change for women and a new sisterhood based on protest and revolt. Many of the writers included are listed elsewhere in our bibliography.

The New Woman's Survival Sourcebook. New York: Knopf, 1975. Paperback. This sourcebook of information for women covers a wide range of issues and information emerging out of the women's movement: work, money, health, lifestyles, children, sports, education, literature and women's culture, the arts, religion, law, men, etc. It includes several pages on mental health, with referral addresses, bibliographies, and journals.

Rich, Adrienne, *Of Woman Born: Motherhood as Experience and Institution.* New York: Norton, 1976. In this extraordinary book, Rich explores her own ambivalent feelings and experiences as a mother and the relationship of motherhood to patriarchal institutions. She raises deep questions and emotions about a woman's mother, grandmothers, self, and children. Rich is widely known as a feminist and a poet.

Rowbotham, Sheila, *Woman's Consciousness, Man's World.* Baltimore Md.: Penguin Books, 1973. Paperback. This book has become a "standard" book in feminist theory. As it describes women's work, housework, and everyday life, it illustrates the feminist motif "The personal is political." Rowbotham, as a Marxist, is concerned with showing the relationship of women's everyday lives to the economic system and with extending Marxist analysis to include the situation of women. The book has some marvelous discussions of how women perceive themselves through the eyes of the dominant culture and how painful as well as liberating it can be to change.

Russell, Dana E. H., *The Politics of Rape: The Victim's Perspective.* This book presents an excellent discussion of the myths and realities of rape, relating the phenomenon to the general mores of the masculine ethos and examining the way rape relates to how women are perceived ("Females as Prey," "Females as Cunt," etc.). Based on in-depth interviews with rape victims, it also describes how women who have been raped feel and the problems they have in convincing anyone of their victimization. The section "Rape and Race" is very good, as is the bibliography.

Women in Transition, Inc., *Women in Transition: A Feminist Handbook on Separation and Divorce*. New York: Scribner's, 1975. Paperback. An informally written guidebook by a women's collective, this book covers a wide range of material from the legal to the emotional aspects of divorce and separation. It includes sections on children in transition, financial and legal resources, insurance, employment, custody, emotional issues and needs, working-class and middle-class women, and lesbian women.

Female Sexuality and Reproduction

Boston Women's Health Collective, *Our Bodies, Ourselves, A Book for and By Women*, 2nd ed. New York: Simon & Schuster, 1976. Paperback. (See also description in "General Books and Anthologies.") This is the best general resource book for basic information about female physiology. The section on sexuality, however, should be used in conjunction with the Shere Hite book, which documents the tremendous variety of female sexual experience.

Brecher, Ruth and Edward Brecher, eds., *An Analysis of Human Sexual Response*. New York: Signet, 1966. Paperback. This book presents an explanation of the Masters and Johnson book, *Human Sexual Response*. It is less technical than the original and easier to read, and it also contains some additional studies in sexuality.

Hite, Shere, *The Hite Report: A Nationwide Study of Female Sexuality*. New York: Dell, 1976. Paperback. Hite surveyed 3,000 women on their sexuality—with questions on arousal, orgasm, oral sex, masturbation, lesbian sexuality, and so forth. The book contains some statistics, but its real importance lies in Hite's taboo-breaking: Hite simply quotes what women have said about their bodies and their sexuality.

Masters, William H. and Virginia E. Johnson, *Human Sexual Response*. Boston: Little, Brown & Co., 1966. If you want to go to the original research that destroyed the two-orgasm theory and for the first time attempted to measure and describe what happens physiologically during human sexual response, read this book. However, the information and methodology are presented in highly technical terms.

Sherfey, Mary Jane, *The Nature and Evolution of Female Sexuality*. New York: Vintage, 1972. Paperback. This book, written in quite technical language, is a useful supplement to *Our Bodies, Ourselves*. It contains a discussion of psychoanalytic theories of orgasms, detailed charts of female sexual anatomy, sexual differentiation of the fetus, and the function of the clitoris.

Lesbian Women

Abbott, Sidney and Barbara Love, *Sappho Was a Right-On Woman: A Liberated View of Lesbianism*. New York: Stein & Day, 1973. Paperback. The first part of this book, "What It Was Like," describes clearly and eloquently the problems lesbian women have in a society whose institutions and cultural attitudes assume that heterosexuality is the norm and lesbian lifestyle is "sick." Part Two, "Living the Future," describes the personal and collective movement for lesbian liberation.

Boston Women's Health Collective, *Our Bodies, Ourselves, A Book For and By Women*, 2nd ed. New York: Simon & Schuster, 1973. Paperback. See especially the chapter "In America They Call Us Dykes," which contains both general discussions of legal and psychological pressures on lesbian women and extensive quotations from various lesbian women on their experiences in a society that assumes heterosexuality to be the norm.

Brown, Phil, ed., *Radical Psychology*. New York: Harper, 1973. Paperback. This anthology contains several articles that relate directly or indirectly to lesbian experience: Jane Coleman's "Surviving Psychotherapy" is a good personal account and analysis of the problems gays meet even with "liberal" therapists. The Radicalesbians' "Woman-Identified Woman" is a clear explanation of how women are psychologically and institutionally "colonized" in a male-dominated society. Carl Wittman's "Gay Liberation Manifesto" is included also.

Brown, Rita Mae, *Rubyfruit Jungle*. Plainfield, Vt.: Daughters, Inc., 1973. Paperback. This exhuberant novel about growing up female and lesbian in a heterosexist culture vividly portrays the destructiveness of traditional sex roles and the prejudices of homophobia; it also presents a strong hero who doesn't commit suicide or go crazy.

Grahn, Judy, *Edward the Dyke and Other Poems*. Oakland, Cal.: The Women's Press Collective, 1971. Paperback. All the poems in this book are important poetic statements of women's experience (especially the "Common Women Poems"), but "The Psychoanalysis of Edward the Dyke" is an especially telling satiric attack on therapists' stereotypes of lesbian women.

Martin, Del and Phyllis Lyon, *Lesbian/Woman*. New York: Bantam Books, 1972. Paperback. This book is particularly valuable for its clear, direct explanation of the repressive stereotypes of lesbians and the wide variety of actual lesbian experiences. It also includes sections on lesbian mothers, lesbian political movements, lesbian sexuality, and lesbian fears.

Women: Racial and Cultural Minorities

Amerasia Journal, special issue on Asian-American women. Spring, 1974. (Write to Asian American Studies, Center Publications, P.O. Box 24A43, Los Angeles, CA 90024.)

Angelou, Maya. *I Know Why the Caged Bird Sings*. New York: Bantam, 1969. Paperback. This autobiographical narrative of Angelou's experience growing up as a Black woman covers more fully many of the aspects explored in the short stories in Washington's *Black-Eyed Susans*.

Asian Women. 1971. (Write to Asian Women's Class, 3405 Durnelle Hall, University of California, Berkeley, CA.) This is a collection of essays, fiction, poetry, and personal reflections, all by Asian women. It covers such topics as "herstory," third-world women, and the politics of womanhood.

Baum, Charlotte, Paula Hyman, and Sonya Michel, *The Jewish Woman in America*. New York: Dial Press, 1976. This book explores the position of Jewish women in America with reference to attitudes in Jewish tradition. Historical information, literary analysis, and a useful bibliography are also included.

Cabello, Gomez and Herrera Cabello, *The Chicana: A Comprehensive Bibliographical Study*. 1975. (Write to Chicano Studies Center, University of California, 405 Hilgard, Los Angeles, CA. 90024.)

Cade, Toni, *The Black Woman: An Anthology*. New York: Signet, 1970. Paperback. This book is a collection of short stories, poems, and essays on Black women. Most material focuses on contemporary Black women, including authors Nikki Giovanni, Audre Lorde, Alice Lorde, Alice Walker, Paule Marshall, and Frances Beale.

Civil Rights Digest: A Quarterly of the U.S. Commission on Civil Rights, Special Issue on Sexism and Racism: Feminist Perspectives. Spring, 1974. This issue contains essays on Puerto Rican women, Native American women, Chicanas, Asian-American Women, and Black women.

Cox, Sue, *Female Psychology: The Emerging Self*. Chicago: Science Research Associates, 1976. Paperback. The section entitled "Ethnic Diversity of Female Experience" contains articles on Black women, Chicanas, Asian-American women, and Native American women.

de Dwyer, Carlota Cardenas, *Chicano Voices*. Boston: Houghton Mifflin, 1975. Paperback. This collection of essays, poems, and excerpts from novels has one section on the Chicana woman in addition to sections on La Raza, El Barrio, La Vida, and La Causa. Of particular value is the selection from Richard Vasquez's novel *Chicano*; see also Marta Cotera's article on Chicana and Anglo feminism.

Kingston, Maxine Hong, *The Woman Warrior: Memoirs of a Girlhood Among Ghosts*. New York: Knopf, 1976. This novel, a combination of the realistic and the fantastic, is a powerful tale of an American-born Chinese girl who must confront both the "living ghosts" from a previous life in China and the new "ghosts" of the Western world.

Koltun, Elizabeth, ed., *The Jewish Woman: New Perspectives*. New York: Schocken Books, 1976. Paperback. This book is a collection of essays, mainly by Jewish feminists, who are exploring the sexism in Jewish tradition, discovering buried aspects of Judaism that hold out liberating potential for Jewish women, and proposing ways to revise the patriarchal aspects of the religion.

La Cosecha/The Harvest, De Colores Journal, Vol. 3, no. 3. This special issue on women includes articles on Chicana writers, the role of the Chicana in the development of the Pueblo Chicano, and papers on the status of women in literature. You can order a copy for $2.50 from Pajarito Publications, P.O. Box 7264, Albuquerque, New Mexico 87104.

Lerner, Gerda, ed., *Black Women in White America: A Documentary History*. New York: Vintage, 1973. Paperback. This book is an important resource for reading first-hand accounts and analyses of Black women's experiences in white America from slavery times down through the present. It has eight articles written after 1960, but its primary value is to give historical perspective on the experience of Black women today.

Martinez, Elizabeth Sutherland and Enriqueta Longauex y Vasquez, *Viva la Raza: the Struggle of the Mexican-American People*. New York: Doubleday, 1974. This historical account of the Chicano and Chicana from pre-Columbian time to the present includes much information on the role of women.

Morgan, Robin, ed., *Sisterhood is Powerful: An Anthology of Writings from the Women's Liberation Movement*. New York: Vintage, 1970. Paperback. (See also annotation in "General Books and Anthologies.") This anthology contains three useful articles on Black women: Frances Beal's "Double Jeopardy: To Be Black and Female," Eleanor Holmes Norton's "For Sadie and Maude," and her "Statement on Birth Control." There is also a section called "Colonized Women: The Chicana" with articles by Elizabeth Sutherland and Enriqueta Longauex y Vasquez.

Ortego, Philip D., *We are Chicanos: An Anthology of Mexican-American Literature in Several Genres*. New York: Washington Square Press. Nine of the forty authors in this anthology are women. The volume also contains a useful introduction, historical backgrounds, and a bibliography.

Rosen, Kenneth, ed., *The Man to Send Rain Clouds*. New York: Viking Press, 1974. This anthology contains short stories by and about Native Americans, with several stories by women.

Russell, Dana E. H., *The Politics of Rape: The Victim's Perspective*. New York: Stein & Day, 1975. Paperback. The section on "Rape and Race" does a good job of introducing the historical context and contemporary experience of interracial sex and rape of Black women by white men.

Vital, Merta, "Women: New View of La Raza" in *Chicanas Speak Out*. New York: Pathfinder Press, 1971.

Walker, Alice, *Meridian*. New York: Pocket Books, 1977. Paperback. Walker's novel centered on a Black woman is superb, painful, and illuminating. It explores the experience of a Southern Black woman in a way that clarifies many of the differences and difficulties between Black and white women.

Wand, David Hsin-Fu, ed., *Asian-American Heritage: An Anthology of Prose and Poetry*. New York: Pocket Books, 1974. Paperback. This anthology contains English translations of Polynesian oral poetry and works by both immigrant and American-born Asians and Filipinos. Only five of the twenty-three authors represented are women.

Washington, Mary Helen, ed., *Black-Eyed Susans: Classic Stories by and About Black Women*. New York: Anchor, 1975. Paperback. This is one of the best sources available on the problems of Black women. The short stories cover such areas as the white standard of beauty, the mother–daughter conflict, the Black family, the Black woman–white woman conflict, and growing up Black and female.

Magazines and Journals

Ain't I a Woman, P.O. Box 1169, Iowa City, IA 52246 $5/year

Chrysalis, The Woman's Building, Department 4150, 1727 North Spring St., Los Angeles, CA 90012 $10/year

Conditions, P.O. Box 56, Van Brunt Station, Brooklyn, NY 11215

HealthRight, Women's Health Forum, 175 Fifth Avenue, New York, NY 10010 $5/individual, $10/institution

Issues in Radical Therapy, P.O. Box 23544, Oakland, CA 94623

KNOW reprints, KNOW is an organization "dedicated to making known the needs brought about by the changing roles of women and men in our changing society." The group has printed or reprinted more than 350 articles, including many on feminism and therapy. KNOW, Inc., P.O. Box 86031, Pittsburgh, PA 15221

Lesbian Connection, Ambitious Amazons, P.O. Box 811, E. Lansing, MI 48823

Madness Network News, P.O. Box 684, San Francisco, CA 94101

Ms, 123 Garden Street, Marion, OH 43302 $9/year

No More Fun and Games, Cell 16 Brewer Street, Cambridge, MA 02138 $1/issue

Off Our Backs, Room 1013, 1346 Connecticut Avenue, Washington, D.C. 20036 $5/year

Psychology of Women Quarterly, Department of Psychology, California State University, Hayward, CA 94542 $3/year

Quest: A Feminist Quarterly, 2000 P St., N.W., Washington, D.C. 20036 $9/year

Second Wave, Box 344, Cambridge, MA 02139 $3/quarterly

State and Mind (formerly *Radical Therapist, Rough Times, RT: A Journal of Radical Therapy*), (See especially issue on Women and Psychology, vol. 3, no. 1, September 1972 and issue on Women, vol. 4, no. 5, December 1974) P.O. Box 89, West Somerville, MA 02144 $6/8 issues

Women and Health, issues in women's health care. SUNY College at Old Westbury, Old Westbury, NY 11568 six times/year; $12.50/year; $2.50/issue

Index